The Fugitive Mind

The Fugitive Mind

the early development of an autistic child

by Peter Rowlands

J. M. Dent & Sons Ltd
London

First published 1972

Made in Great Britain
at the
Aldine Press · Letchworth · Herts
for
J. M. DENT & SONS LTD
Aldine House · Bedford Street · London

ISBN 0 460 07876 3

Introduction

The eldest of our four children, John, is autistic. His handicap is milder than many others', but unfortunately very real. He will probably never seem completely 'normal' to people—(whatever that means)—but we feel certain now that he will seem more so the older he gets. Over the past three years he has made a great deal of progress. Before that there were times when he seemed to be drifting further and further away from other people.

Few agree on what is the most important part of childhood in which to learn to do things. If you have a child who is consistently getting later and later at developing what other children pick up quickly, you try to find out about critical learning periods, and what it means when they are missed. This is difficult because 'late normal' can mean all things to all people. Some years ago, when we finally learnt what was wrong with John, we read, and we were told by a child psychiatrist, that the age bracket four to six can be crucial. This is a period of which it is sometimes claimed that speech must be learned then, because it will only be gained in a very rudimentary form later. Happily, this view is from time to time disproved. But over the past years it has been impossible for us not to think of it. You can't put it out of your mind.

When John was seven (and this book was completed) it did not seem that he had much time to spare. But, thank God, it does at last look as if the groundwork for his future has been laid. He has started to talk; to play with other children; to get on with the world like other little boys. And he has become all the happier for it. A big transition began during these years, although every year of his childhood is going to be important.

When I heard John's diagnosis, and became convinced of its truth, one comforting idea occurred to me. If I started noting things down, *then*, there would be some kind of record of these years that might help other parents who found themselves in this strange territory. Whatever the outcome, some other people might be given a better idea of what to expect, and at least a feeling that they were not utterly unusual.

We ourselves didn't find much to read that gave a parents' eye view. There were some books and articles that were informative, challenging and helpful in that they forestalled any hopes we had of a quick cure, or of an educational system that would take care of John's main needs in training. The good ones are mentioned in this book. But the rest were uniformly depressing. My message is that John is doing well. Not magnificently well perhaps, but well enough to make us very happy and excited. I hope this helps.

It took a long time for us to reach the point of saying to our doctor, 'We are worried sick. We *hope* he is just slow. But it seems as if there is something basically wrong that is holding him back. For God's sake, get us an appointment to take him to a psychiatrist.' If there is any possibility at all that your son is normal, you don't want to reach this point. But in the end, when your doubts are too big to submerge any longer, there is a lot of relief to be gained from going to an established authority and asking him to say what is what. He speaks, and at least he will take the doubts away.

But if your child's mind is fugitive and eludes understanding, doctors, clinicians, psychiatrists will often disagree. And if they can't agree on what is wrong for him, it is unlikely they will say the same things about what you should do for him. The same child can be called 'normal, but emotionally disturbed'; 'mildly autistic'; 'schizophrenic'; 'sub-intelligent'; 'maladjusted'; 'symbiotic'. All are sometimes flags of convenience. Some imply a theory about causation, some don't. This is not something for which you can round on the psychiatrists. No two children with mild handicaps are exactly alike. And they are often different children on different days; at home, and in the consulting-room. After a while you are tempted to think that your child must be a kind of freak because no one can decide about him.

Knowing about other parents, through mental health societies, helps get your own problems into perspective. For us it meant realizing that there were other children who were like John, more or less, and that there were certain kinds of things that could help them to be happier, and to start learning what would be useful to them later. No one who reads this book is likely to have a child that fits John's pattern perfectly, but anyone who sees similarities may get a feeling that his own child is not alone. He may like to see how one family has adapted to the presence of a handicapped child in the household: this family has been happy enough, with plenty of compensations for the problems.

There are three questions that must affect every parent of an autistic child. 'What is autism?' 'What causes it?' and 'Does it exist as a single definable handicap in its own right?' I don't pretend to go near to answering them. These are things which other people often expect us to know. But they demand full-time application from doctors and psychiatrists before definite facts can emerge. I am neither. At the same time, since the answers to these questions affect my wife Pat and myself about as much as anything else in life, I have made it my business to discuss the concept of 'autism' and its causes. This is limited to practical observations within the book itself, and the results of reading about the subject and discussing it endlessly. In an Appendix I've prepared a fuller account of current medical thinking on autism. This can be missed out if the reader prefers to stick to John and his doings, and avoid the technical terms.

Parents of autistic children form a minority group. A survey in Middlesex suggested there may be about five thousand families in Great Britain with an autistic child. This would put autistic children midway between the numbers of children who are deaf and those who are blind. Both these latter groups have, rightly, well-developed educational facilities in this country. Autistic children, by and large, are not nearly so lucky. Much is being done, but it takes money and time, both of which are at a premium—especially critical learning period time. I feel strongly about this, no less so because John has proved luckier than most. If anyone gets the impression while reading this book that autistic children will *repay* greater effort in developing educational units for them—quite apart from humanitarian considerations—then writing it will have been worth while.

John, Louise and Simon

This reference page shows John's progress, on a time-scale, so that it can be compared with that of his sister and brother. It can be used to check how old each child was at different moments of the story.

	John	Louise	Simon
1962			
	Born		
1963			
	Age 1 'Bottom-shuffling' Singing begins (wordless)	Born	
1964			
	Age 2 Stood; walked		
	Reciting poems Toilet trained	Age 1	
1965			
		Walked; ran	
	Age 3 Reading began 1st diagnosis		
		Talking began	
	Definitive diagnosis	Age 2	
1966		Reading began	
	Age 4		
	Speech: about 10 words	Toilet trained	
		Age 3	
1967	Began school at T	Nursery school	
	Age 5		
	Speech: about 50 words	Age 4	Born
1968			
	Age 6		
	Began school at S	Began school	
		Age 5	Age 1
1969			
	Age 7		
		Age 6	Age 2 Walked; talked Reading began

Chapter One

Pat was with John in a waiting-room at A hospital. There was a long wait while the consultant worked through the other mothers and children in the queue. Nobody talked much, except when trying to keep their children quiet. Pat had this problem just as much as the others. John was nearly four, but could not be told anything complicated about what was going on. She couldn't say to him, 'Wait just a bit more, and it'll be our turn after that little girl over there.' He had not the slightest idea what he was doing, or where he was, or why they were waiting. Small wonder that every now and then he would pace heavily along the line of chairs, and look for something interesting —another child's toy, a pen on the nurse's desk, a door handle.

'John! Come on, come and sit down.'

He could respond to this, although this afternoon his patience was wearing very thin. He knew his name; and he knew what to do when you asked him to stand up, sit down, eat his breakfast and so on. But very rarely, if ever, would he say anything in answer.

Pat's way of keeping him quiet had to be rather different from the other mothers'. 'Let's say "The Owl and the Pussy-cat", John.' He smiled, without looking at her, and intoned the whole poem. No stops—he never needed any memory-jogging. And as far as *he* was concerned there were no mistakes. He had the rhythm and the sound of the words almost perfectly. But here and there he had caught a word imperfectly from us, and once it was stuck in the flow of the poem it stayed there unchanged. '. . . By the Turkey, who lived on the Pin,' he used to say. The turkey went on living on a pin for ever. Whether the bird was comfortable or not made no difference to John. Because, with the arguable exceptions of 'Pussycat', 'nose' and 'hand-in-hand', not a single word meant anything to him whatever.

When it was over he soon got bored again. This caused him to 'gurn'. A 'gurn' is a noise that is exactly what it sounds like. Being nasal, and wordless, it grates on the nerve-ends. It is always threatening to reach a climax, which is best avoided since it brings explosive screams of rage.

Another thing Pat could do to cut short the gurning was to sing to him. By now she was quite used to doing this among strangers. John would smile, and be very good—provided the singing was not too long. Sometimes he joined in himself, although he was past the point when he sang at his best.

They went into the consulting-room at last. The consultant said, 'Hallo, Mrs Rowlands', and 'Hallo, John'. Then he watched as John ignored him completely, and went straight to a gleaming silver torch on the side of his table.

'Can you make it work, John?' the consultant asked quietly.

John didn't touch the switch at all, again ignoring his voice. He was more interested in the glint of the light coming from a lamp in the corner of the room that spangled on the surface of the glass.

There were a lot of questions the consultant had for Pat. But he reserved most of his attention for John. No doubt it helped him make an assessment, but it also made sure that his torch remained intact. At one point he showed John how to switch it on and off again. Pat's heart sank. Our son was now utterly fascinated, and, sure enough, howled with rage when the torch was finally taken away.

'I'd like you to bring John in for a couple of days, if you don't mind. There are some tests I'd like to make.'

Luckily this was a hospital with a strong sense of duty to obey the spirit of the Platt Report. This meant that Pat was allowed into the children's ward with John, sharing a small double room with him. For a couple of days he played with the toys in the ward, while from time to time he was withdrawn to have his heart checked, his urine tested and his brain waves scanned by EEG. An X-ray photograph was taken of his brain—rather blurred, Pat gathered, because he got very impatient with the time they took. He was even persuaded to yield up a small sample of his blood, although he fought the nurse with the needle right up to the end.

On the evening of the first day the consultant visited Pat in the little double room. He looked at John, who was asleep. 'He really *is* a handsome boy,' he said.

We've always thought so, naturally, and we've often been told so too.

'What do you think is wrong with him, doctor?' Pat asked. 'Have you reached a decision?'

'Well——' He paused, and studied Pat with the attention he had hitherto reserved for John. 'What do you think yourself? Have you any theory about him yourself?'

Without thinking—the answer surprised her later—Pat replied, 'Well, yes, we felt he might be a little autistic.'

'Yes, I'm afraid he is.'

This was it then. The two watched each other for a while.

'Do children *stay* autistic?' Pat demanded at last.

The consultant spread out his large hands and studied

the hole between them. 'There's not very much known about autistic children. Severe cases—John's is not like that at all of course—have to be hospitalized. Others get along—some better, some worse. Some do quite remarkable things. . . .'

He looked at Pat as though rather surprised that she was taking this situation so calmly, without any obvious emotion. In fact she felt a curious sense of intense relief. It was as if she had been screwing up her eyes, staring at a ball balanced on a knife-edge, for several years on end. Suddenly it fell. On the wrong side. But at least it fell.

'How do you——? What causes it, exactly?'

'Nobody knows very much about that. There are one or two books you might get hold of. I'll write them down for you. Meanwhile I'd rather like to see you again, in a week or so. Could your husband come along too, do you think? And John's little sister?'

'Yes, of course. How far—do you think John will get?'

The consultant turned his eyes towards John's face again, pressed tightly to his teddy-bear. 'He *is* handsome, isn't he?' Then he turned back to the space between his hands. 'It's very difficult to know how these things will turn out. If we watch the next three or four years carefully . . .'

Which is what we have had to do. And partly to make it easier for other parents to know what they might expect—partly because John himself seemed to deserve being written about—Pat and I decided to make notes on what happened.

But first it seems sense to start John's story at the beginning. I have written down the main details about his birth, his illnesses and the first impressions he made on us. This kind of detail may turn out to be more significant when people know more about how autism is caused. But it all provides a background to our state of mind at the time of the diagnosis, and to the reconstruction period after that.

Nothing occurred at John's birth to make us think that there could be anything wrong with him. He came about ten days late, which is by no means unusual for a first-born child. There had been a 'false alarm'—again, not unusual—which meant that Pat was in hospital for nearly eighteen hours before delivery. The labour itself took less than four hours. Gas and air were refused by Pat, and she had a pethidine injection instead. This was in line with the Lamaze instructions she had received in a course for expectant mothers run by the National Childbirth Trust. At M maternity ward she came across one midwife who was rude and unsympathetic, succeeded by another (luckily, just before delivery) who was friendly and efficient, and willing to put extra pillows under Pat's back when it ached. The doctor was a student from Nigeria: he was thoroughly understanding, and gave the impression of being thoroughly competent too. There was no tear during labour, but an episiotomy was felt to be necessary.

Everything seemed to have happened more or less according to plan. Pat was happy and confident when John appeared at half past four in the morning, weighing seven pounds, fourteen and a quarter ounces. 'No abnormalities' was recorded on his labour record sheet. I myself was unable to get into town to see him until half past eight. By this time Pat was feeling much too happy still to be thinking seriously about trying to make up for lost sleep. The first thing I saw, entering the ward, was a grin from ear to ear on her face. I sat on her bed, while John was brought in and placed between us. He seemed to have perfect features, except that while the top of his right ear curled over, the top of his left ear was flat. It was as though this part of him hadn't *quite* had time to get finished. He had very dark eyes and a thin sprinkling of dark brown hair.

John's attitude was rather more puzzled, rather less belligerent, than most new-born babies we have seen. There was something about him that suggested he needed re-assurance about the kind of world he had come into. 'It is a strange place, baby,' one of our friends commented to him when she saw him. At the same time we had absolutely no grounds for thinking that he might be different from others in any essential way.

Nor was there anything in the family history, either on my side, or on Pat's, that would have prompted us to be alert to the possibility of something odd in our children. Longevity runs on both sides, with rheumatism or rheumatoid arthritis the only physical conditions that affected more than two near relatives. Pat's father had died of TB—but his working conditions must have contributed quite as much to this result as any hereditary predisposition. If we had no qualms from a physical point of view we certainly had none on the mental side. Two of my blood relations have had nervous breakdowns, but these were brief and their recovery was firmly based.

We had had to wait longer than we wanted to have our first child. We were twenty-nine and twenty-eight respectively. There were one or two alarms during pregnancy itself. In the eighth month Pat slipped on some icy ground and fell. But this had no discernible effect on the baby's activity—he kicked fairly often to remind Pat he was there. At the antenatal clinic at M hospital some comment was made on the fact that the baby had assumed an unusual position in the seventh month. But two doctors, at successive visits, had different views on this; and, at any rate, for three weeks before birth John had manœuvred himself into a perfectly normal upside-down stance.

During the week that Pat remained in hospital after delivery John received a lot of attention from the nurses. He was a sort of favourite among them, and they all—the English, the Irish, the West Indians and the Spanish—commented on his being 'a very good-looking baby'. He seemed to have got international approbation at a very early age.

Feeding started without any trouble. He took to the breast after a little coaxing the first time, but didn't need the lesson repeated.

We don't know what tests were made on him at M, but certainly nothing was mentioned to us as worth keeping an eye on. No one suggested anything special by way of diet. Leaving the maternity ward, he was confidently expected to sweep all before him.

When he was brought home, to a new house we had just started to buy, we were entirely happy with our new family, and looked forward to the days when he would start showing us what kind of character he was going to be.

Neither Pat nor I had had any young children before to look after. Pat had had short spells as an au pair in France and Spain, it is true, but hadn't been asked to attend to babies. Quite possibly if we had had younger brothers or sisters while we were still at home—or, of course, if we had had a child of our own before—we might have noticed certain odd differences in John, or become curious about them at an earlier stage.

He did not take long to prove he could smile. And in due course he demonstrated explosively how he could laugh. He liked to be pleasantly surprised—being shown a new toy, or by daddy making a funny noise—and he adored being tickled. While he was enjoying himself he seemed totally happy.

He cried a lot too. It suited him to have his food at particular times, and he was loud in his anger if he didn't get it quickly. When he needed winding or changing it was the same. But there were frequent times when, despite being well fed, dry and winded, he still wanted to cry. What we learnt from our next two children made us feel that he cried a lot more than other babies.

At the time there were lots of reasons we could think of, and worry about too, for this crying. He could be cutting some very early teeth, or he could have a sore throat, or earache, or some terrifying new disease that would shatter the medical world. All kinds of possibilities passed through our inexpert minds. Cuddling didn't help a great deal when he was 'well away'. He enjoyed being held and talked to quietly sometimes, but usually only when he was in a good mood to start with. What did help, dependably, was rocking; or, better still, being pushed in his pram.

This was sometimes a doubtful advantage. After a difficult morning Pat found it very pleasant to plant John in his pram and propel him to the shops. The movement kept him happy—just so long as it went on. Some shops had wide enough doors and no steps, so that he could be kept moving. Elsewhere he had to be left outside, and this he would not tolerate. Some shop assistants realized that it was better, quieter, to help Pat through her shopping as quickly as possible. For a period he became suspicious of any hesitation that Pat made, to look into a shop window or to talk to a friend, just in case it meant that he was going to be left still.

There was one morning when she had to visit a particular shop with a narrow entrance, where the pavement outside was too cramped for her to leave the pram. John was parked outside the grocer's next door—and then she got caught in a slow-moving queue. When at last she got away she found the pram empty. Up and down the road there was no sign of John. Then she saw him, through the grocer's window, in a policeman's arms, towards the back of the shop. A passer-by had been convinced by his cries that he must have been abandoned indefinitely. The policeman had been summoned and he was now investigating the matter. Pat noticed, thoroughly shaken as she was, that the policeman, too, was finding it difficult to keep up a constant rocking motion for John and scribble his notes at the same time. The shock of seeing the empty pram took a long time to wear away.

Suddenly the demand for movement came to an end. We don't know why. It simply didn't seem to matter any more. There have been a great many other things that John has insisted on at different times during his life. They have developed very quickly and disappeared just as mysteriously. One thing doesn't necessarily take over from another. In each case John has shown himself to be very anxious to preserve something, often unimportant to others, but obviously crucial to him, for much longer than a normal child would wish, or even tolerate.

Another way of calming John down, from very early on, was to give him some music. This became more important to him later, when he was a toddler, but his pleasure in music began very early. It didn't matter whether it came from a concert on the radio, or children's records on the gramophone, or even from our own voices. It didn't take us long to notice that his temper improved rapidly as soon as it started.

But, despite his periods of crying, the main thing as far as we were concerned was watching him growing bigger and enjoying the sun more. Being born in late March gave him the advantage that he could be put out of doors early in life, to take the air and the sun, and to get brown without running the risk of catching cold. For a long time he was free from any kind of physical trouble, major or minor.

If we had had more experience, then perhaps we might have made more of a peculiarity that in fact we only appreciated in retrospect. Whenever either of us came up to him, looked at him and made noises, he might or might not smile, but usually his eyes would pass away from ours, and his gaze would be on our shoulders, or farther away still. It wasn't that he turned his head to one side. (Had he been obviously trying to avoid us, we would certainly have taken more notice.) It was as if his eyes were drifting to one side, rather unwillingly, refusing recognition, but with some regret. At times we felt he might be bored with us; or tired; or registering annoyance; or looking to see if there wasn't any food around. Whatever it was, it seemed a superior thing to do, not a sign of weakness.

Once more it was easy enough to rationalize what was happening in the comments we passed to each other. It was a mild source of pride that we had a son who apparently didn't need a constant interchange of glances with his parents. 'He's a bit disdainful this morning, isn't he?' one of us might say to the other. Or, 'He's suspicious, isn't he? Wonders what I'm after.'

Years later we were to meet a lot of autistic children with 'fugitive eyes'. John's 'non-look', though not as marked as most of theirs, might have told us something if we'd known what to watch for. At this time, though, why should we have worried? He was big, healthy, strong-looking and handsome. You only had to bounce him up and down on your knee, or tickle him, and he would react delightfully. Again—without looking you directly in the eyes.

Chapter Two

John was a long time sitting up. Since he was so big and solid, it seemed reasonable to wait until his muscles felt more like supporting him. At about nine months this happened. This was well within the normal range, although some might think he was cutting it a bit fine. What was less normal was that he never actually crawled. Once his first birthday had passed he began 'bottom-shuffling': that is to say, he would sit up, place his hands to the right and left of his knees and propel himself forward. As he did so his bottom shuffled across the floor. More than once it occurred to us that if we dressed him in a dust cloth, it would do the parquet a lot of good.

For a whole summer and autumn this was his sole mode of progression. Other friends' children had sometimes done this at one time or another, but never for very long. John had a very solemn, purposeful look when he was doing this. He made you feel that he knew his own mind, and had deliberately chosen this method.

One of my great-uncles claimed it was traditional for males in his family to say 'I won't be druv' whenever the womenfolk made too many demands. They would then be like mules, sitting down and ostentatiously doing nothing. There was some heredity coming out here perhaps.

The first time we went on holiday as a family it was to a Cornish seaside hotel. John was coming up to fifteen months. He did many of the things babies do at the seaside.

He found sand interesting to grind between his teeth; he found that sitting in the sun by a rock pool, scooping up mixtures of sand and water, was a nice way to pass the time. He adored being carried by mummy or daddy as they ran into the waves. But he showed not the slightest interest in other children. It was a family hotel, so there were a lot of children to choose from if he felt particular about whose advances to encourage or turn down. For a while toddlers would come up to him, put one of his toys in his hands and make friendly noises.

Then, in the end, they lost interest.

There was a swing in a field next to the hotel garden. One afternoon we put him onto the seat, held him by the shoulders and gave him a gentle push. He was shown how to clasp the upright chains and enjoyed it rather solemnly. But when we took him off he howled. We put him on—he stopped. We took him off again . . .

During this holiday we discovered just how relaxing it can be to have responsibility for a loudly crying baby in an hotel. Many meals we abandoned because as soon as John had had all the breakfast or lunch he wanted he shrieked his disgust at waiting for us to have our fill. But the nights were far worse.

In the small hours we were convinced that every other person in the hotel, and maybe the annexe too, had been roused from sleep by the noises coming from *our* baby's cot. We groped towards him in the dark, murmured songs and pleaded with him to be quiet. At breakfast we felt everyone must be glaring.

On dull, rainy days John was very difficult to please. Then we found a table tennis set in a games room. We hoisted the net, got bats and a ball. A sulky John was put down in the corner of the room and we started to play. We didn't get very far. As soon as he saw his parents cavorting at either end of the table, making curious batting sounds against the ball, he exploded with laughter. It was so infectious that we had to laugh with him. He shuffled across to us, a great beam on his face, to get a closer view. This was when, in fact, he really mastered the bottom-shuffling act. Any attempt to play the game properly soon meant jumping or tripping over our son, who kept on breaking out with laughter at us. Once we realized that neither of us could hope to win it was a thoroughly enjoyable game.

Coming back from that holiday it occurred to us that we had seen a lot of other children and none of them was very like John. They were all ages of course, but this was our first opportunity to see children en masse, close to. Neither of us said much about this to the other until several days after our return. It seemed somehow disloyal—until we found that the same vague thoughts had occurred to both of us.

We had realized that John was holding back in a lot of things. He said nothing whatever, except for occasionally repeating the word 'bear' when we said it to him. This referred to a large teddy-bear, who meant a great deal to him, and had been a night companion ever since he was three months old. We often called John 'Bear', because his shape suggested it, his constancy of expression underlined it and 'bear' was all he said. We still use the name sometimes.

Nor did he show any sign of wanting to stand up. In his cot he was willing to be stood on his legs, and to be held while his hands were placed on the rim of the bars, and he would stay there for a while. But it was not until he was fully one and a half that he levered himself up alone. As he was large and heavy we worried about his sending the whole cot crashing over as he struggled with one side of it. Play-pens he would never tolerate.

His eyes would still move away if we wanted to look into them. We knew now that he did this with other children just as much as with us or with other adults. We alternated between talking about his 'not being very sociable' and wondering whether he ought to have his sight tested.

Meanwhile down the road from us a little girl who was born one week earlier than John was running around and chatting away to people. She was much closer to what we imagined most other children of his age must be like. From now on looking at other people's children often brought us a jolt, despite the fact that we had read Dr Spock on the subject of comparisons and saw the general wisdom of his point that they should be avoided or ignored.

Then again, if he had been behind in *everything* it would have been much easier to observe, and admit, that something was wrong.

In fact John was consistently ahead of his age group in toilet training. He was very intolerant of being wet or dirty. Early in his second year he quickly learned that Pat was delighted if he produced something at the moment when he was undressed and sat down on the pot. He seemed to like the regularity of the arrangement—and of course it suited us to suggest that he might produce at regular intervals. He was never told off if he refused to co-operate in this on any occasion, or if he had an 'accident'. Whenever he was caught unprepared he made it quite clear to us that whatever we felt about it he himself was furious. In course of time he showed that he could use the lavatory by himself, and could remain dry at night. He achieved all this earlier than his sister.

Again, at eighteen months, he could build a tower of coloured bricks to a height above his head. He looked almost smug as he shuffled round it on his bottom, surveying it from all sides. The only nuisance was that if such a tower fell over or was disturbed he could sob and scream for a long time. Sometimes it spoilt his temper for the rest of the morning.

Music seemed to charm him more and more. And before his second birthday he could already sing, wordlessly, in tune. This meant a great deal to us. The purity of his voice at this age always brought us a special thrill that no other music has been able to supply before or since. He didn't always want to sing; we felt honoured and very delighted when he did.

What did it mean? What would happen, we wondered, if we had a young genius here who might want to compose piano sonatas at six? How on earth could we, who enjoy but know little about music, help him properly?

The idea that he might have some special musical gift must have owed a certain amount to wishful thinking on our part. But it was strengthened by the fact that it did not seem to matter very much what music we played for him. Mozart or nursery rhymes, he listened, rapt, just the same.

But, gift or no gift, there was surely no need to worry, we told ourselves. If his mind was capable of registering music and getting it repeated, as well as of building up a perfectly respectable set of toilet reflexes, we felt that his brain must be basically sound. He preferred music to language, obviously. Well then—who was to say he was entirely wrong?

But although we were concluding these arguments satisfactorily and optimistically from our point of view, we had arrived at the point when it was already necessary to argue it through. This was one stage in the growth of our doubt.

Victoria (the little girl down the road) seemed alarmingly quick and responsive whenever we saw her. She was always bright and friendly—she looked up at you pertly, and asked what you were doing. One Easter Sunday the difference between her and John suddenly became cruelly sharp.

They were both just two years old. I was walking back from church with John, and saw Victoria with her father crossing the road to visit us from the other direction.

'There you are, Victoria,' I heard her father saying. 'There's John and his daddy.'

Instantly she was skipping ahead of him towards us. Much faster than John, I noticed. She was bubbling over with laughter, very excited. A small white package with a blue bow was held precariously in the crook of her arm.

'Hallo, John! Hallo, Mr Rowlands!' she cried. 'I've got an Easter present for John!'

She thrust it under his nose. 'Here you are, John,' she said, more quietly and very winningly. She was still hopping up and down with pleasure.

John looked briefly at her, at the present and then beyond them both. He was completely impassive. Then he turned abruptly at right angles, and walked straight up to our door without a word.

'Oh, John!' I cried.

Victoria was very close to tears. She let me take her present for John, and then went back quietly to her father to talk it over.

'Honestly,' I remember saying to Pat afterwards, 'we've got a stubborn character here. He's just a curmudgeonly old bear!'

She laughed. 'You can almost see him saying to himself, "I won't be druv".'

This is the sort of way we protected ourselves, without actually knowing about it, from harsher interpretations. About this time we started explaining to other children, 'John's a bit shy, you know,' so that they would not take against him.

There was another situation that might have meant more to us than it did at the time. Twenty months after John was born, while he was in bed, Pat gave birth to Louise at home. Again taking advice from Dr Spock I had bought a blue railway engine, just over two feet long, as a 'birthday' present for John. I led him into our room, where Louise held court, puffy and swaddled and half a day old, kept tightly at Pat's side.

He took not the slightest notice of Pat or Louise, but his eyes seized on the train immediately. He pulled it clear of the bed, sat down and pushed it on one side. The wheels had shiny hubs, and he soon became engrossed in the patterns they made as he spun them round. There was a bell behind the smokestack, too, which he felt needed testing. When I lifted him up to show Louise to him he looked round anxiously for the train. It wasn't for several weeks that he went up to Louise of his own accord: to poke at her, and give her a good smell.

But if I had to sum John up at this time it would *not* be that he avoided people—which is the rather superficial comment often made about autistic children. He was delighted with attention from us as a rule. Sometimes he would be so taken up with a toy, or something in the street, that he would ignore any person near by. And when someone was being especially introduced, as with Louise, he usually found something else to look at. Yet it was by no means a simple matter of rejecting all advances from living beings.

One important element in his life was Bristol, our Siamese cat. This was an intelligent animal who had a highly developed sense of play where John was concerned. Two things John loved to do—to smell Bristol, and to feel his face close to his fur and rub it gently. Most of the time the cat allowed this quite happily. John also got the idea of throwing something along the floor for Bristol to chase and bring back. This was delightful to watch, and not in the least what you might expect from a handicapped child.

His need to smell and to feel things though, might, with hindsight, have given us a clue. For many autistic children these senses sometimes seem to be almost as important as sight and hearing. When John first saw our new lawn-mower there was no doubt in his mind what he needed to do first—he shuffled over to it and sniffed pensively at the motor. I disliked his inhaling petrol fumes, and tried to draw him away. But my father said, 'What would you *expect* a bear to do?' Then we let him satisfy his curiosity in his own way.

Quite a few people besides us were making comparisons between John and other children. But they always found it very difficult to talk to us about this. Mostly they were unsure of their ground. What did it actually *mean*, for instance, that John said very little, except for a word or two, or a line from a song, which he repeated often? What conclusion do you draw? Do you say that he's preoccupied; a slow beginner; spoilt; unfriendly; lazy; eccentric; unsure of himself; over-cautious; anxious? Do you go further, perhaps, and suggest that he must have something wrong with him—bad metabolism; brain damage; psychogenic disorder? Against this, at the times when John was two, three and four years old, there were the facts that he looked very handsome; that he developed impeccable toilet training; that, although he was slow, he learned to walk and run well enough; that he was uncommonly musical.

Looking back, Pat and I have a lot of sympathy for those friends and acquaintances who suspected something was wrong but didn't want to say anything outright to us. There was no reason why they should hurt our feelings, or worry us, if they couldn't be sure they were right, and couldn't be sure what they were right *about*.

We must have put them off too. We are certainly as proud of our children as anybody, and sensitive to any possible criticism of them. One of the results of the way we were brought up and educated has been to make us unwilling to accept what anyone advises, whatever authority they are supposed to have, without carefully examining it first. We are, possibly, over-cautious about accepting others' opinions on matters that are inside our normal 'territory'. Moreover I myself did a degree course in psychology. How were they to presume that here was one cobbler's child who was badly shod?

There was a similar kind of problem in communication with the local clinic. The doctor there once recommended that John should have a hearing test. When this showed, however, that his hearing was as acute as anyone would wish no further doubts were expressed. But one day a health visitor came around to see Louise and was struck by John's manner. Without knowing what was wrong she felt that she needed to discuss her misgivings with the clinic doctor.

When Pat visited the clinic some time later, for Louise's benefit but with John in tow as well, a pointed question was asked about John's lack of interest in what was going on. But it wasn't followed up, and it merely succeeded in making Pat defensive.

Anyone who saw John casually at this time was much more likely to be impressed than anything else. His photographs show that we haven't just stored up an idealized view of what he was like. At two and a half he was tall, with a straight back. He looked solid, purposeful, self-sufficient. His colouring was dark, except for his cheeks which were usually rosy, healthy looking. Long dark eyelashes formed a defensive ring for his eyes. The eyes themselves were a strange mixture—blue on the outside, brown on the inside.

His hair was very dark brown, and perfectly straight, except for a duck's tail at the back. He had perfectly clear skin—never spotty, and always looking as if he had just come back from holiday. But what was most striking about him, perhaps, was the way in which he seemed to have perfect symmetry. There was a sense of balance about his face—there still is—that made you feel that every feature had been carefully weighed and measured before it was attached. Only the tip of his left ear, as we had noticed at his birth, suggested a tiny flaw.

When he moved, even, there was nothing very odd to strike you at once. It took observation to notice that he moved rather slowly for a child his age; that he never made quick running movements except after a certain solemn deliberation. He was learning to come or go as you asked, but needed time to consider how to translate your request into what he should do with his feet. And when he had to pick up or hold something he seemed uncertain which hand to use.

His voice was, at this age, extremely musical. The more so to us, perhaps, in that we didn't hear it saying anything very often. Singing, he seemed to have perfect pitch automatically without trying. If they heard him sing people used to feel he must be a sort of show-off who was basically rather shy, because he ignored their compliments and would not answer their questions.

Temperamentally he struck you as being not easily aroused, phlegmatic, self-sufficient. He enjoyed things like horse-play, but expected them to come to him rather than to show that this was what he wanted and give us a cue. But when something went wrong for him that he really minded, he could howl and throw tantrums with the best of them. And there were his 'off-days' on which he would wander disconsolately from one part of the house to another, gurning and finding fault with everything. A child psychologist, the wife of an acquaintance, paid us a visit on one such day. Her comment was that John 'will be much happier when he can talk and tell everybody just what is wrong'. I am sure there was a lot in what she said; what proved to be the case, though, was that his inability to understand enough to be able to learn to talk was precisely what was wrong.

Chapter Three

John came into speech via music. For a long time there was nothing but 'bear', as mentioned before. There was later also 'no'—which he used liberally for a while without seeming to care whether he started or stopped anything by saying it. When other children might have been saying 'Mummy', 'Daddy', or 'Hallo', he was struck by the sound of 'Three Blind Mice' on a gramophone record. He intoned 'Dee Die Dice', but was much closer to the tune and the rhythm than to any of the other words.

We were offered an old piano, which we took in mainly for Pat to play in the evening for the children before they went to bed. This was a difficult time as John and Louise were usually both over-excited on being taken out of their bath. John could lose himself completely in the playing and the singing. Any bad temper slipped away by magic. Louise showed a pert curiosity in what was going on, but was back to her toys if the music went on too long. Nursery rhymes were the mainstay of each concert, together with a set of children's songs from different countries. But John had shown a liking for a wider range of music, and Pat extended the repertoire for him. Tudor madrigals delighted him especially. For days he went about chanting his own version of Henry VIII's 'Pastime with Good Company'. His uncompromising look certainly suggested a stubborn Tudor streak.

It did not take long for this bed-time sing-song to become

a ritual. Soon it was not *we* who were deciding on it—it was John. Any suspected delay would have him jumping up and down with impatience. Whenever we were late, and felt like putting him to bed without his usual music session, it took a lot of tact and persuasion to avoid a violent showdown. We had built, if you like, a system that took charge of us. But it was good to see John completely enjoying something we gave him. This was the one way in which we could get directly onto the same wave-length with him and stay there for any space of time.

That summer holiday, then, meant that some travellers on Western Region trains had the doubtful pleasure of listening to Pat calming John down with a song or two whenever the length of the journey began to tell on his temper. If anyone in the carriage glared we told ourselves that the glares would be far worse if we ignored John and he really let fly.

Some of the songs were French, so possibly we were dismissed by some fellow passengers as quaint foreigners who needed to be humoured. By accident we had found a series of French children's songs on records. John was enraptured by them. He insisted on hearing them over and over again. They were more successful with him, perhaps, than English records. This has been explained to us since as an indication that he was autistic. The reasoning is this: an autistic child cannot understand language, feels the pressure on him to learn it and resents it; therefore he appreciates something far enough removed from ordinary language (for example, French) not to recall that pressure. This is as it may be. But other children like the French records too, and I believe they do so because the French tend not to 'sing down' to children and so they sound more genuine.

Louise soon realized that there were record sleeves with pictures on that related to the songs. So she studied both *together*, getting a story out of what she heard, while John attended only to the sounds that he liked so much.

It was very exciting for us as more and more words, and lots of phrases, came out of John's mouth as he joined in singing. The best moments were when he was not prompted but simply came out with part of a song while walking round the house. Soon, he seemed to be promising us, soon he would be giving us real speech. At moments like these it was difficult not to believe that speech was just around the corner; and that all we had to do was be a little more patient and it would come.

I was a late talker myself as a baby. One day, at two and a half, without warning, I looked at my mother and asked, 'What are you doing that for?' Apart from 'Daddy' and 'Mummy', and various obscure noises, these were apparently my first words. Why shouldn't John be like that too?

That same holiday Pat and I stayed at a cottage in Somerset. We were on our own and one morning, while washing up, Pat tested the resonance in the kitchen with 'Voi che sapete' from *The Marriage of Figaro*. Much later in the day, John gave her back the first sixteen bars without any hesitation whatever. Later that summer, at home by the piano, he showed that he could sing it right through, after practice, just with piano accompaniment. He could do this alone, but he seemed to prefer singing with someone else. A cue word or note pleased him—possibly because this was an active reminder that the song was something that we did together.

Music was all very well, but even child prodigies have to talk sometimes. He seemed to be getting a better idea all the time about what we wanted him to do—('Hold out your hands so I can put on your gloves . . . thank you, John')—but he wasn't transferring much from music into talking or everyday life. This was not just because of Mozart and French songs either. He liked 'Mulberry Bush', and we thought that 'This is the way we wash our hands' might start to mean something, gradually, in a bathroom context. But there didn't seem to be the right kind of bridge.

So we took one of his birthday presents, *Apply Dapply's Nursery Rhymes* by Beatrix Potter, and read them to him. There were lots of animals we could point to in the book when their names came up. There were lots of simple words that must, we felt, be useful to him very soon.

It took some time before any of it started to click with him. It wasn't that he didn't enjoy it—he liked attention of any kind, even if he moved off quickly once he had got it. When we read to him, though, he listened to the sounds with an air of somebody being patient. He looked at the pictures too, both scornfully and vaguely at the same time. 'Are you trying to tell me this nonsense is important?' he seemed to be saying to us. It was difficult not to feel we were being humoured. He really wanted to be picked up, turned upside-down and tickled; or taken outside into the garden, and rolled down the slope towards the apple tree.

Then one afternoon as I carried him round the garden on my back, murmuring the rhyme about 'the amiable guinea-pig', John joined up with me on

> 'He wore a sweet tie
> As blue as the sky . . . '

It doesn't sound much, but it was wonderful. It had been a long time coming, and it seemed a big reward.

With normal children, certain milestones are of course important—first walking; first time he's dry through the night; first complete sentence; etc. Most parents are pleased when their child reaches them, and they feel proud. But you notice very little things if you have a very slow or a handicapped child—the first time a word is spoken properly; the first time a button is done up; the first time he draws a man's face, and puts in the eyes. Even minute improvements in the extent you feel you are 'close' to him—often without being able to say why or how—can make all the difference between a happy day and a wonderful day.

Despite this triumph there was one lingering disappointment with that holiday. On walks we raised John up alongside the brown and black noses of some horses, who wanted us to provide sugar lumps. But these, and tractors, sheep, farmyard dogs and even strawberry plants, seemed to leave him absolutely cold. Other parents were having a fine time showing these things to their children for the first time. We were missing out for some reason.

It didn't take John long to build on the 'amiable guinea-pig', until he could say the whole set of poems through with us. He was pleased, and proud of himself.

When he was having an off-day for some reason—either because Louise was badgering him for things he couldn't understand, or he wanted things that he didn't know how to ask for—he would make noises at us and say the first line of a poem over several times. This he would continue until he got us to go through it with him. This was frequently an easier way of calming him down than putting on some music or singing. It still must have seemed odd to some people, though, seeing Pat, John and me chanting our way through nursery rhymes together while Louise murmured what sounded more and more like the real thing.

We tried reading John stories, but they obviously meant nothing to him at all. Occasionally we would strike a story with a rhythm or rhyme to certain lines, which would seize his attention. When you reached, for example,

Little pig, little pig,
Let me in! Let me in!

he would laugh, say it through again, and show not the

slightest concern about whether or not the wolf got to blow the house down, or eat up the little pig. You could go on telling the story, but he was still on the short piece of poetry in the middle. It was like a jam tart to a boy who hates pastry—you might just as well give him a spoonful of jam.

So we tended to go back to Mother Goose, Edward Lear and Lewis Carroll. He had his preferences, although he was prepared to lend an ear to most of the poems we tried. 'The Owl and the Pussycat' was a special favourite. He proved this by saying it together with us, right through, the third time it was read to him.

At first we couldn't quite make out what it was that struck us as odd. Then we realized, unmistakably, that while *we* still needed to refer to the book John didn't really need *us*. Looking back, I'm sure he had practically every syllable by heart after two readings. I must say 'practically', because he muddled a few of the consonants—hence the turkey being condemned to live on 'the pin' instead of the hill.

His vowel sounds were a bit odd. Many were perfectly normal, but others he produced with a kind of sing-song tone, almost as if he were mocking himself. Sometimes he said words lazily as if he could only be bothered with those syllables that appealed to him. He sounded a bit like a foreigner who has got English intonation nearly but not quite right.

Any letter in combination with 's' was liable to give him trouble. Many children do some sort of lisping, but usually it disappears after a while, and often only a few sounds are affected. With John it is *still* there now. 'Looks' used to be 'loosk' when he first said it. Now he sometimes over-compensates and says 'looksk'. When this started we seemed to have a Russian bear in our family.

Whenever we heard him start up long poems on his

own—even in a supermarket, where anyone must have thought us odd—we didn't want to put John off his recital.

We had lost out on requests that other children make of their parents from very early on: by the time he was three, and still not talking except in poems, the last thing was to refuse to recite with him. This was John, doing something clever, and offering us something. It came much closer to normal contact between parent and child in the average family such as we were then beginning to enjoy with Louise. When it means this much you encourage it, even when he is calling through the lavatory door to begin again.

Perhaps we overdid it: I don't know. On the one hand you can say that it helped him get used to saying things, and that this helped the more useful, meaningful language to come later. At the same time it might have made him so satisfied with a sort of sterile language that it may have delayed his coming to terms with the need to use language actively. Anyway, we can't change it now.

And I'm afraid we showed off with our close friends and relatives. They were becoming wary of asking us, 'And how is John now?' They had stopped making suggestions like, 'I expect he's running round, playing all sorts of games with his friends, isn't he?', or 'Chattering away now, is he?' Instead they now asked simply, 'And how *is* John?', meaning that they would like to ask more, but they didn't want to embarrass or discourage us. Suddenly there was something John could do, to give them a reason for revising any poor opinion they might be forming. Maybe he didn't say hallo to them, or answer any questions he was asked, or behave like other little boys of three, but when had they last seen a three-year-old who would recite several sizable poems, at a cue from Pat or myself? It was further proof for a time that John had tremendous potential, of a kind that we couldn't quite appreciate as yet. There was nothing much wrong with him, but there might be a lack of understanding in ourselves.

As he spoke more and more poetry it was a great mystery for us how much he could actually understand—or, rather, how many words or phrases had some kind of meaning for him, over and above their place in the poem.

'Hand in hand' was obviously a useful phrase for John to appreciate if he could possibly grasp the idea. Sometimes we would repeat the words as he reached them in 'The Owl and the Pussycat', holding out for his hand at the same time. On the roads, where he showed not the slightest understanding that there was any kind of danger beyond the kerb, we repeated 'hand in hand' again to him—sometimes rather desperately. In the end he accepted the cue: if you said 'hand in hand' to him in an insistent tone, it meant he should meet you half way and put his hand into yours. It took a long time, and this fact in itself gradually convinced us that not much sense was being derived from what he learned.

It was curious that as he recited more the pure tone of his singing seemed to fade. He still enormously enjoyed music sessions around the piano. But he was more content with humming rather than imitating the sounds of the words; and he compressed tunes into a narrow band of notes. Rhythm was coming to be more important to him than melody.

He was taken to play groups at three. It was not easy for Pat to watch the other children learning to play together while John was barely at the stage of learning to play at all by himself. There were mornings when he had to be held in her lap if he was not going to scream. Sometimes he would go to the door, stamp and shriek with rage at anyone who tried to close it, and watch it with great intensity as he slowly turned it through an angle of ninety degrees and back again. He could do this for hours.

Music at the play groups wasn't always provided. If Pat volunteered herself, and there was a piano to hand, John could in fact be charmed off her lap, or away from the door, and he would enjoy it with everyone else. He refused to sing with the other children, however. And when these children were being taught their first singing games he kept well to one side.

As he got more used to the children's presence, and what they did, he became intrigued by the patterns they made. Eventually he could be persuaded to join in and start with the others, going 'In and out the dusty bluebells', but it was never for long. He would slip away and make for the side of the room, just as you thought that *this* time he was well and truly in. From this refuge he would cast glances back at the others from time to time—at the magic circle he could not join. These were suspicious, disdainful and envious looks all at the same time.

The mums who were there too would smile knowingly and say he was shy; he would soon get over it. Pat, however, knew that she had been using this excuse for much longer than the start of the play groups.

A strange reaction he produced at another child's birthday party intensified her doubts. Because children did not become friendly with him—and, probably, because other parents found him odd—the number of birthday parties John was invited to got fewer as he grew older. We were delighted whenever he got an invitation; later we worried, in case he did anything that would rule him out from going to the same house again. But any invitation for John became like a rich, unexpected present. On this occasion we hadn't bargained for what would happen when they started 'musical bumps'. All the other children paced, jigged or jumped, with a look of determined rivalry in their eyes, waiting for the piano to stop. Several made false starts at sitting down. John just stared at the piano, delighted. For them the music was a means to an end. For John it suddenly gave the party a purpose.

When it stopped, then, he made a beeline for the piano, and roared his disapproval. Bumps, children, winning a prize, meant nothing. Starting and stopping a tune in the middle struck him as being no more than a particularly nasty form of teasing. Pat took him into the kitchen to let the others get on with their game.

This kind of thing became much easier to understand later. At the time it was just a puzzle. The explanation that it showed how stubborn he could be had worn thin. But, with hindsight, what John did at that party was something entirely natural for him, which we might have predicted had we been wiser. We know now what a birthday party must have been like for him. First, there was a strange house with a number of children—some recognizable, some not. He didn't know why they were there, or what he was doing there. Being in a house with one other child was one thing. But parties must have been a wild jumble. Bringing a present along was just to have something bright and shiny put into his hand, only to be taken away. At the party itself there was food. That he could understand: only illness could put him off his food. He was usually the first to arrive at table and the last to leave. Not just greedy—this was a piece of living that fitted into the jigsaw that he knew. Apart from that there were instructions he could not understand. He became confused and had to be pulled this way and that during games. Why on earth should he try to join in? The idea of competing too, of beating the others and winning prizes, meant absolutely nothing. So why get entangled in these strange activities, where the rules seemed to change every five minutes? Wait! Here's some music though. That's different! Suddenly the pattern of sounds reaching him *becomes* a pattern, and it forms a protective shield against the turbulence of the voices. When it stops . . .

He had his own ideas about what was musical and what was not. When we visited an uncle who had a budgerigar in his living-room, John came out violently against bird-song. Haydn's Toy Symphony, with its tin whistles and other nursery noises, seemed to cause him acute pain. 'In a way it's such *sad* music,' commented my cousin when she saw him whimper and hold his ears at the beginning of the slow movement. This showed what a strong sense of choice John could make other people feel he had. We were taken in ourselves at first, but Pat remembered how he could take against bird noises, against train whistles, against the car's squeak when grit gets into the disc-brakes—it's all in the Toy Symphony.

Similarly he was very pleased with the early passages of Smetana's *Vltava*. The young brook, the peasants dancing, the nymphs in the moonlight—fine. But the waterfalls and the battle made him feel he needed to protect himself from the wild, crashing chords. We had to be careful about the records we put on for him.

Since that time, when he was three, he has got used to makeshift bands, with tambourines, cymbals, drums and triangles. He is less fussy about noises he doesn't like, but he has become less likely to be completely engrossed in any new music.

His tastes took on a boyish tinge. At Christmas, when he was getting on for four, he had *Peter and the Wolf* as a present. Peter's tune was nice, and he would hum it with us. But not so nice as the 'shooting' of the kettle-drums, when the hunters were firing through the woods. Even now he still doesn't know what a gun is, but it sounded exciting. 'Bang-bang!' he shouted. I raised an eyebrow. Pat made me lower it again. 'Exactly what a little boy should say,' she told me.

Chapter Four

Most mornings John would come into our bedroom just as I was starting to shave. He seemed able to judge the time perfectly. He came straight over with a vague 'Mm-mm' of greeting. He watched me carefully as I wetted my face, rubbed the shaving stick against it and brushed up some lather. When I worked over my left cheek (the side away from him), he held my knee and craned round my body to get a better look. I was being inspected to make sure my preparations were complete. As soon as I'd finished with the brush he started to chant, in an insistent sing-song, 'A-meh-meh-meh-mo! A-meh-meh-meh-mo!' I would dot lather on his nose, which used to amuse him. Usually I just let him take the brush, which he put cautiously to his cheeks, and then into his mouth to suck. Provided I took a reasonable time with my razor he didn't mind when I took the brush back to wash it.

Except that most boys don't care for the taste of soap, this is perhaps unexceptional. But John enacted every detail the same way every morning for about two years. Occasionally Louise came too. Not to be outdone, she also cried 'A-meh-meh-meh-mo!', and spread lather over her cheeks. But she could take it or leave it alone.

It didn't stop in the morning. There were rituals right through John's day that had to be observed. We supported many of them on the grounds that he liked routine, and life was much easier if we all followed it.

A short while later in the mornings he would observe me putting on my contact lenses. This used to alarm me at first—thinking of a quick grab for the lens container, or for the precious disc on the end of my finger as I was raising it up to my eye. But I soon learnt that he had no such intentions. His part came later, when I had to let him put on the container's two screw caps, one at either end. These were coloured white and blue. It occurred to me after a while that I might get him to distinguish between the colours. 'Now the *blue* one,' I said, putting the blue one in his hand; 'now the *white* cap.' Soon he didn't need assistance. And in the end he himself said, 'Now the blue one,' etc. . . . What we did not know at the time was that his idea of 'blue' and 'white' was restricted purely and simply to lens container screw caps: he couldn't generalize and pick out a white feather or a blue balloon.

Of course it couldn't be exactly the same every morning. If I overslept, or had to go to the office early, he sometimes missed the lens ritual. Then he would rush round the bed to where I was sitting, crying 'Cap on! Cap on!' If I didn't get the container back down off the shelf, unscrew one cap and allow him to replace it solemnly, it soured him for the whole of breakfast, and beyond.

The final touch was to put back the container in a particular position in the wall cabinet. Both children liked being appointed to this task, since it meant my picking them up. They had to take turns, which was a difficult concept for John to grasp.

'No, John. Louise's turn now,' was something we had to say to him, as in this case, to defend her interests while she was still small. The words made an impact on him, and they were played back to us, in one form or other, for some time. 'Louise's turn!' he sometimes shouted when angry and when something was frustrating him. Often it had nothing to do with Louise at all. One summer afternoon, after ice-creams in the garden, John dived at the lurid wrappers that had been tucked under a deck-chair. As he clearly intended to eat these as well they were taken from him. Disgusted, he stamped his foot, and cried, 'Louise's! That's Louise's turn!' Louise turned her head from the paddling pool to see what she might be missing.

But following him through the day again—after putting away my lens container he allowed his dressing to be finished. We believed in trying to get both him and Louise independent in this from early on. If sweaters were back to front sometimes what did it matter? John learned to do simple buttons at three and a half, shortly after Louise first mastered one (she was just approaching two at the time). Top shirt buttons are still difficult for him now, at seven, and the buttons of his shirt sleeves he simply cannot manage. Shoe buckles he managed very creditably at five. These had to be learnt in two stages—and on one of these he actually beat Louise. Shoe-laces he tangles, without success. Up to the time he was four, then, there was a certain amount John could get on with, but there were odds and ends to be tidied up. This was my job most mornings, after which he expected me to say 'Hand-in-hand' and walk with him down the stairs to breakfast.

One day I counted the stairs out loud, which he liked. This had to be repeated for a long time, and he joined in with relish. Numbers were never used for anything else but stairs, except for an abacus—on which a visiting relative once got him to count up to ten as he rolled the beads along.

Downstairs in the kitchen some minute details had to be correct if we were to survive breakfast without shattered nerves. He had a particular stainless steel spoon that any new au pair girl found tricky to tell apart from the others in the drawer. If this was not beside his cereal bowl in the morning he would look round as if we had insulted him. 'My size spoon!' he shouted, or words that sounded very like that. While Pat or I fumbled in the drawer, the sink or behind the fridge, his roars of 'My size spoon!' got more threatening, and sobs crept into his voice. This demand lasted about eighteen months.

Shorter, but much worse for us, was a strange habit he picked up just before he was four. He decided that the only way to sit down at table was to start with the chair pushed right in, about six inches from the table edge. The chair had then to be absolutely straight. He saw it as his task to sidle into his seat, clutching the table top to keep his balance while he bent his knees forward. Every morning we waited nervously for this rite to begin. Sometimes he managed it first time, but far more often he nudged the chair out of line before he considered himself properly seated. This meant gurning; then rage. It was useless popping pieces of toast in his mouth or even singing to distract him. We learnt, painfully, that the harsh rules he had set himself simply had to be followed. If his temper broke down completely during these efforts we took him into the sitting-room, where he could listen to a record before coming back and trying again. We had about six months of this before it stopped completely, as mysteriously as it had begun.

The rest of John's day depended more on us. If Pat went shopping she usually took him along. Or he stayed in the house and played by himself, pausing for food, records, going to the lavatory. There was a ritual component in most things—such as always playing with the swing doors at the supermarket.

As soon as Louise's coming was certain we started having an au pair girl in the house. We insisted, when we made arrangements with each new one, that she should stay a year, or at least ten months. This way we felt the children wouldn't feel that there was always someone coming or going.

Our very first au pair, Ingibjorg from Iceland, had a young nephew who could run around at fifteen months, converse fluently at eighteen months and feed himself entirely independently at two years. We were informed of his progress each time she had a letter. The gap between him and John became so wide that she realized we did not appreciate this running commentary.

But Ingibjorg took to John, and spent a great deal of time sitting down with him, exchanging toys and noises or simply watching. She respected his rituals and was very loyal towards him. If she thought we were wavering the least bit in our confidence about his abilities she could be sharp in his defence. 'He's not stupid, you know!' she flung at me once when I commented gloomily how long he was taking to start talking.

When some big change happened we anticipated the worst. Changing au pairs, moving house, going on holiday—we always suspected this kind of thing would really disturb him. But the big changes never did. He seemed curious, bemused perhaps, when he left our house one morning to stay with friends for a few hours while a furniture van took everything away to our present house. When he was brought here he looked round, making little fuss, ate a good tea, bathed with Louise as usual and had a good night's sleep. It was the same when Ingibjorg gave way to Bjork, and Bjork to Ireen. So there was a new face at the breakfast table—so what?

But if he couldn't find the toy car he was currently interested in, or if he found the catch was stuck on a door he liked to open and shut, it was an entirely different story. People and things were all spread out on a scale of importance that was utterly individual to him. We had to learn this scale, because it was quite unlike our own. We had to subscribe to many of his values—by helping him mend the windmill that always came apart, by waiting for him to touch each lamp-post we passed. Sometimes it was too much: he had to be ignored or we would miss a train. Or he had to be picked up bodily and carried into the bathroom, despite all screams, or he would never get to bed. I don't know whether we gave in too often or too rarely. Certainly his rituals often fed on themselves—that is to say he found something mildly interesting, repeated it, then found it irresistible. Maybe we should have nipped some of these off. But if he was *enjoying* something, unless our tempers were near breaking point, it took a stern outlook to stop the fun.

A pleasanter side to his need for ritual was that if Pat or I were doing long, repetitive jobs in the house or the garden he was happy enough to be with us, watching the ironing, or the weeding, or, better still, the lawn-mowing. It was good to feel his companionship as he walked up and down, next to me, as I worked the motor mower across the grass. At the end of each swathe he liked to dart forward, as I turned the machine round, and peer at the bits of engine that he could see vibrating. 'John! Get back!' I shouted at him. But in fact he could judge the angle of its turn very accurately, and he always kept out of harm's way.

The best part of gardening was when I had been hard at it for an hour or so, vaguely aware that John was around. Suddenly I would feel him clasping me round the back from behind. Then he would either take my hand and guide it towards a hand-fork that he could use close to where I was working, or he would start to sing or recite something. He did not offer his company like this easily or regularly, but when it came we felt ourselves honoured.

When he didn't join us we sometimes worried. He was quite capable of going back to the sitting-room from the garden on a bright day and lying down on the settee. 'Dropping out' like this really did seem unnatural. Pat would watch him carefully for other signs that he might be sickening for something. But it was simply a matter of his preferring to keep to himself for huge chunks of the day. He had sociable days and drop-out days. All children change moods—but not this much surely. We felt more and more that there was some kind of invisible curtain that came down between us every now and then.

When the rubbish heap in the garden got too high, and it was a dry enough day for burning off, I tried to get this done while the children were not around. It had only taken one bonfire to make it clear that everything about fire fascinated John. The flames and the crackling of twigs made him jump up and down, edging closer and closer. He gave no sign of having the slightest idea of danger, and I was forever pulling him back. But the smoke, it seemed, attracted him more than anything. He could stand for about ten minutes if you let him in the middle of a thick stream, his eyes wide open, breathing it in, glorying in it.

On a bonfire day the very suggestion that we wanted him back indoors for tea made him howl. He had to be carried back, the length of the garden, while he flailed with his legs, straining to get free. Little specks of ash filled his bath, and his clothes smelt as if they had been hanging for a week in a chimney.

It's much easier now to look back at what John was like at three and fit the pieces of jigsaw together. At the time we saw the differences in his strange behaviour, but failed to notice *similarities* in the kinds of things that made him different. Not having been given the diagram to look at, we didn't even know that here was a jigsaw puzzle at all.

We were still waiting for him to catch up—to reach a stage that wasn't going to come.

All the time he was trying to find patterns of meaning. This is easier to understand with music, perhaps, since this was a straightforward substitution: instead of a jumble of sound he opted for a tune. Poems served the same purpose, to reorganize meaningless noises into a predictable stream. Standing in the smoke hardly seems to come into the same category. But it does if you assume that not just sounds but all bodily sensations are confusing to him. This would mean that a sensation as all-enveloping as breathing in smoke achieves the effect of shutting out the confusion, because it is consistent and forces concentration on one thing. Splashing rhythmically in his bath may have had a similar effect to standing in smoke, although once more the basic sensation was utterly different.

Rituals are more complicated. But if the patterns of sounds in speech are unintelligible to an autistic child it makes sense that each day, or a morning even, must seem very strange to him. It must seem like one inexplicable thing after another happening in no particular order—unless the autistic child takes it upon himself to give some structure of his own to it. The same things, then, need to be done at the same time, in the same way, day after day. That way life can start to make sense.

It is reasonably easy, then, to understand John looking for nice rituals which he could keep going happily. But why should he have become anxious to sit down in the same peculiar way every meal time? This operation was so difficult that it was deliberately courting the danger of failing at it which threw him into a tantrum. Such a ritual makes much less sense.

But the principle behind the rituals may be the same, even though each one may vary in being pleasant or unpleasant.

To put it simply, we suspect we know why the ritual game is being played, although we find it difficult to follow the rules.

I believe that in most of what John did—and in what he involved Pat and myself in doing—he was trying to make sense of a strange world. Why it should have been so strange for him is still difficult to understand, even with our hindsight. There were perhaps three main reasons. First, and probably most important, he did not perceive things, hear things or generally sense things in the same way that most other children do. Secondly, he had not got the same kind of motivation as the rest of us. For example, it has simply never been important for him to compete with his sister, except when she has taken or obstructed something that he needed for ritual reasons. This could be a part-reason for his concentrating on all sorts of little things that others disregard and ignoring important ones, like the sight of a bus approaching fast. Third, he developed an odd set of emotional reactions. The commonest of these is perhaps just a lack of definite reaction: ignoring the friendliness of newcomers, being oblivious to the worries of the rest of the family and so forth.

This is perhaps too much theorizing at this stage. But the past is always demanding explanation, for reasons that I will go into more carefully later.

'Why can't we have a boy who sits down at table in an *ordinary* way?' Pat once demanded in exasperation. At the time I probably grunted into my coffee. But we have been busy looking for serious answers to the question ever since.

Chapter Five

John has taken a long time to get started. Louise has been on the move ever since birth. Their lives, their doings, their feelings, have been so different and yet so bound up with each other that Louise needs a chapter to herself.

A few hours after his birth John wore a concerned, rather vulnerable, look. Not so his sister, who was red and very puffy from the speed of her entry on the scene. It was not long before she roared for food. Rapidly she learnt that she could staunch her impatience for a while by sucking her thumb. When she rolled her eyes about she seemed to be saying 'Well? What have you got to offer me then?' And John's gentle new-born-baby cry, with its pure tone, became a vague memory: here we had a screecher who sounded like rusty nails.

It took us a month or so to realize that this brash, self-sufficient character had pretensions to charm as well. When the puffiness went, despite the fact that she was bald, she could smile very sweetly. Gradually she was demanding less and smiling more. The big difference was that here we had a baby who was curious about us all the time. Her eyes followed you round the room. When you caught them in a look they stayed there, holding yours, and usually twinkled because she was grinning.

'Look at the way she's lifting her head and staring at us!' Pat once commented with delight to a friend.

'Ye-ess,' was the doubtful reply. She was happy to indulge

maternal pride, but surely Pat must know that *all* babies did just this.

Of course we didn't know this. We had to find out all about babies again with Louise.

While John had been listless a lot of the time, either sitting still or crying but not doing anything to help himself, Louise was energy personified. She raised her head early, sat up early, crawled early and appallingly quickly. She tottered to her feet before twelve months were up. By this time she was prattling things that soon turned into recognizable words. I don't remember her beginning to walk so much as beginning to run. If she wanted something she launched herself impulsively at it—whether it was a teddy-bear, or corn flakes, or me. She seemed to fall over eighty times a day without ever coming to harm.

Our world was too small for her. John had never strayed outside the front garden or shown the least interest in doing so. Louise found, when she was just two, that she could persuade her brother to push upwards on the 'up and over' garage door to give her a gap large enough to wriggle through. One hectic morning she was at last found, clutching a carrier bag, two hundred yards and two street crossings away. An adult stopped her and asked her, doubtfully, what she was doing.

'Going to the shops!' Louise replied and strode purposefully by.

After this scare we over-reacted by having all sorts of padlocks, bolts and iron bars attached to any door or window that she might use in order to break out. The house felt like a maximum security prison.

Her nature was so utterly unlike her brother's that it may be wondered why we didn't conclude immediately that something was wrong with him. But it seemed natural enough that we might have two children with different personalities. Later it also occurred to us that we might have one very bright and one moderate, but not abnormal, child. Of course we clung to the first interpretation as hard as we could.

Louise had never known what it was to have a brother who competed with her—until Simon was born, which was not until she was nearly four. John was a very nice sort of brother to have in many ways. A less determined child might have found him dull as a companion and would have stopped, or cut down, contact with him. Not so Louise. She chivied him into taking notice of her, and established a very close bond with him. She did this by drawing him, often forcibly, into any game she wanted to play.

At first it went like this. She would notice that he had something in his hand—say a friction toy car. She would crawl up to him and jog his elbow. Sometimes she seized the car, but more often than not she was content to make him do something with it, together with her—be it only tug-of-war. John would then find his hand guided to the floor, and then moved up and down, to get the friction toy working. Even before she could talk she could make a noise that clearly meant 'Now let it go, John!'

Obviously he was often unwilling to join in. But although he was twice her weight she was the quicker. Moreover she was always persistent, and seemed to know as many ways as a cat does to get what she wanted.

There were days when she presumed too much on his temper. He was curious to watch when this happened. Suddenly, fed up with her fussing him, he put down what he was carrying, faced her squarely, drew breath, planted his large hands against her chest and pushed. As this could send her half way across the sitting-room we didn't encourage it. When Louise picked herself up, burst into tears and came over to us of course we comforted her. But we usually added, 'Well, you see—that's because you drove him too far.' By trial and error she worked out what John would stand and what he wouldn't.

Although she wanted her own way, this usually meant pleasing John as well as herself. Pat observed that a happy afternoon for Louise included at least some time in which John would be happily involved himself. Louise needed a companion, not just somebody she could manipulate.

Meanwhile John began to need her attentions more and more. As he grew older he was less satisfied with his own company. Moments when he liked to watch other children, even when he didn't play with them, got more frequent. Louise was the one he wanted to be with. Not the noisy children in the play group who did all sorts of things he couldn't understand. Louise was different: she would come up to him, make him sit down on the floor and say, 'Now, John, see-saws!' Holding his hands, facing him, she would get him to rock backwards and forwards. This was the way to bring him into things, naturally, and without imposing efforts of understanding.

He grew to depend on her taking him by the arm and leading him into whatever mischief she was planning. They got on particularly well together in the sand-pit in our garden. She would decide that all the sand-pit toys—the buckets, the plastic cups, the old saucepan—should be filled with wet sand and decorated like cakes, or with daisies as if they were flower-pots. John had a bucket put into his hands and he was told to fill it. She half pulled him, half cajoled him into getting it right to her satisfaction. It made him very happy. He often made it last beyond the time that Louise wanted to continue. Usually in the end she left John to put the finishing touches to what they had been doing. He stayed in the sand-pit, solemnly filling buckets, turning out the contents, smelling them, decorating them.

In one sense Louise was a systematic destroyer of John's rituals. If he was deep in something repetitive she was likely to bound into the room, crying: 'Come on, John! You've got to be ill in bed, and I've got to be the doctor and take your temperature.' He might protest a bit but his patterns for life tended to crumble whenever she came in: few of them could survive her onslaught.

He was forced to accept her as a peculiar part of the world's system, a joker that he would find in his hand of cards from time to time. She was what a computer programmer would call a 'randomizing agent'. She could be almost relied on to intervene, break up the flow of time, give him new stimulation, change what he wanted to do. So it was important to him that she should be there. When children came to visit us Louise was delighted to play with boys and girls who had fresh ideas for games. She played with them, and John followed at a distance, watching, but unable to join in. He looked philosophic during this. The way he reacted when Louise came back to him showed how much he needed her to 'randomize' his world. When she was taken to nursery school, at three, he made it plain that something very important to him was missing in the house. He wandered from room to room, gurning sometimes, not exactly looking for his sister, but clearly hoping that she might reappear. 'Louise is at nursery school' meant nothing to him for some time yet.

Sometimes Louise imitated the odder noises that John produced, but she quickly gave them up. Talking presented very few problems for her, although sometimes her desire to tell us things outstripped the speed at which she could think of the right words. Once she learnt a new phrase it stuck.

Music and poetry she enjoyed together with John. She insisted, in fact, on not being left out whenever she saw us starting anything with him. But she was more quickly satisfied than he was, and he was often left with us half way through a record, a sing-song or a recitation series. For her, repetition was unnecessary for learning, and she certainly surprised us with the bits of knowledge she picked up apparently without effort and brought out of storage at appropriate times.

They have become very fond of each other. But, naturally, they have had fights. Often this came about when Louise misjudged the importance to John of a particular ritual he was engaged in, when she tried to drag him summarily away. The other main source of trouble has also been mentioned already—John's lack of understanding of the business of taking turns. If she was on the swing he wanted to be on it too. Later she wanted her turn back. He resisted. She screamed. We intervened as referees, as parents always do. The difference was that we couldn't clearly explain the justice we were dispensing.

In any case their fights didn't last long. They were never physical struggles, for the simple reason that Louise soon knew the odds. She knew that although her brother never had the slightest interest in hurting anyone he was strong enough to throw her into the next garden if he really had to.

Louise has always had a very short memory where quarrels are concerned. She was, when very young, the sort of child who can burst into tears, and a few seconds later be rocking with laughter, the tears still flowing down her face. She bore no rancour—and John bore none back.

During the time that I am describing, that is up to the time when John was four, and Louise was two and a half, there was little reason for her to perceive that John was unlike other older boys. Later she became puzzled to find that other boys were not like her brother. But at this time we ourselves were still not prepared to draw a clear line between John and normality. During these years Louise had a splendid companion, though he was in some ways more like a large, amiable, walking teddy-bear than an elder brother.

She was in for two shocks. The first was that other children are not so malleable, not so docile. The second was that her next brother was going to compete for her toys and for our attention with the best of them.

John's co-ordination problems have been mentioned before. It was hard to tell what was wrong exactly. He was tall, strong-looking, with a straight back—but slow, hesitant in his movements and far from agile. Was he lazy? Was it just that he did not understand the point of being quick, of learning to ride a tricycle, of catching and throwing balls? Or was there a weak chain of command from his brain to his arms and legs? This sideways looking that he did—was it a part of general bad muscle control? Or, even, partly the cause of it? We puzzled a lot. But Louise meanwhile improved his performance in all things. So doing, she put our minds at rest again—for the time being.

Louise helped mainly by getting him excited and concerned about doing things in an effective way. At first John took no interest in jumping. Even to get him to run I had to pretend to chase him, crying, 'I'll chase you! I'll chase you!' which he answered by repetition—'I'll chase you!' —and by moving away quickly to avoid being tickled if I caught him. Not that he disliked being tickled—but he judged from Louise that it was something to run from excitedly.

Louise got him to stand on a step outside the french windows, where she would shout 'Jumping!' and launch herself impetuously forward. Her knees were covered in cuts and bruises, but she was irrepressible. John caught the spirit of imitating her, overcame his caution and jumped too. While she did it as if she were brushing off a fly, he gritted his teeth as if he had to do it to save his life. As he got more practice he jumped with his feet together, instead of apart. If he fell over it put him off for quite a time. But Louise would coax him back to it in the end.

The very fact that she might seize his toys if he did not look out helped him to develop a turn of speed, and to use his hands to hold what she wanted above her reach.

Wrestling appealed to Louise too. Once they saw some on television: by mistake, because we'd left it on. Instead of being worried by it, as I'd feared, they both fell about with laughter. Neither used to react much to anything on the television screen, but when one bald monster seized another and hurled him to the ground they thought it was a tremendous joke. As soon as it was turned off Louise leapt sideways into the air, coming down with a bang on the flats of her hands. John copied her, and soon they were grappling on the floor. It continued in the garden, off and on, for a long time afterwards, whenever Louise felt like it. It may sound strange, but it was a relief to see our son enjoying a fight.

She brightened up his bath time by grabbing him round the waist and pulling him, then pushing him, through the water. This showed him he could send tidal waves smacking into the taps at the end. It made him very difficult to get out of the bath. Here too Louise gave him a lead, by showing how to jump from the rim of the bath to the mat below.

She could help him physically more easily than she could extend his use of his mind. He picked up words from her certainly. These he repeated, sometimes aptly, sometimes not. But he was stuck with a few words, while she was acquiring many. He watched her playing with jigsaw puzzles, and imitated her passably. He took some of the simpler jigsaws and did them over and over again. Louise was soon bored with one that she had mastered a few times. We couldn't afford to keep up with her taste for more and more difficult ones.

It seems ungrateful to point out that while she gave him so much, and made his days a lot happier than they might have been, she was limited in how much she could teach him to use his brain. It is even possible that she may have put him off some kinds of learning, through absolutely no fault of hers, but simply by sprinting through new intellectual tasks.

We always felt she was bright, probably above average. Later, when she could read like a nine-year-old at four, we felt she must be well above average. Eventually we took her to an educational psychologist for an intelligence test. The report indicated that she was far ahead of her physical age in a number of things and might need special schooling.

Although he could not possibly have had a nicer sister, it may have been disconcerting for John to watch her grasping new things so quickly. Talking, drawing and understanding associations might have been easier for him, at times, had he had a less clever one. Her patience was limited, just as ours was: if explaining something to him became tedious she left off.

Even before we had two children Pat and I were clear on one thing. If either suspected that the other was devoting too much attention to one child, then this had to be said out loud, and corrected. We both knew it was a danger, and we both wanted to be objective about it. When Louise came there is no doubt that the novelty of her verve tickled our imagination more than the daily puzzle of John.

It was all too easy to build houses and bridges with her for an hour or so; then we would look up and wonder where John had got to; we would walk round to the sitting-room, and find him half sitting, half reclining on the settee, staring at nothing. John soon lost interest in anything constructional that was at all difficult or required an effort to picture what sort of thing you were trying to make. Dividing time between them, or finding things for both of them to join in, was much more of a job than we'd feared. The more so with the gap between our two children getting wider.

What was Louise like, then, at two and a half? Rather small for her age, with very bright blue eyes that seemed as if they could register every conceivable emotion, in sequence, in a matter of minutes. She had golden hair, turning into brown, which Pat allowed to grow long. Around the house she was like quicksilver, throwing herself at anything that caught her eye. Violent changes of mood and temper made an afternoon with her anything but dull. She had a talent for mischief, and for organizing her brother into it. When we heard toys being thrown through the nursery window onto the garage roof, only John was still at the window when I charged into the room: but a guilty look from above the sheets soon convinced me who had instigated everything. At the same time her affection knew no bounds. She would rush to Pat, to me, to John, to the au pair—and embrace each one for no apparent reason, with no apparent message, except for her love.

She was curious too, and addressed herself unselfconsciously to anyone she met. If we took her on a train journey she was as likely as not to say to the old lady in the opposite seat, 'Hallo, girl!' And if she saw someone dozing off in the compartment—'Sleepy? Going to sleep?' She was so natural, and free from any fear or embarrassment, that it seemed a shame, later, to have to warn her about talking to strangers.

Medically she was strong, but in a wiry way, as opposed

to John's more solid frame. She was more prone to coughs and sneezes, and about twice as likely to have a runny nose on any particular day, winter or summer. But she was far from fragile: however many times she tripped over and bumped her head she always picked herself up, ready for the next headlong lunge.

As her voice grew less sharp and jagged, more rounded and more calculated to please, Pat and I complimented each other on what good company our daughter was. She was the most delightful person we could conceive, to talk to in the house, to show new things to, to play with on the common. I must admit she knew all the routes, both direct and indirect, into my good books. She was efficient, yet kind, in the way she managed her parents.

Chapter Six

John was almost always in the best of health. One week, however, he was distinctly below par. It was nothing one could easily recognize. Simply, he went straight to the settee after meals and put his head on a cushion; then he wandered listlessly round the house, picking up a toy only to drop it a moment later, and making gurning noises. His bowel movements were suddenly white. Our doctor could only advise us to watch him and see what happened. Everything remained just the same, except for the gurning noises, which became louder and more nerve-racking; we saw the doctor again, and he made a second examination. This time Pat talked about John's diet. The doctor was struck by her telling him that in addition to sausages, ice-cream, and so forth, John had a passion for margarine, butter, anything that came from the cow, and soap. (Washing his face really meant preventing the flannel from being taken into his mouth and chewed reflectively.) Once he found a quarter pint of double cream on the kitchen table: it took him about fifteen minutes to eat every drop, without being sick afterwards. The doctor suspected a metabolic difficulty, such as a failure to break down fat, so that John took in an inordinate supply of dairy products. He gave us a letter to the consultant at A hospital.

This was the first time Pat went to this consultant. On this occasion she had still to learn how important he was to be. As with most hospital visits with young children the appointment time was only an approximation. After a long wait John was not an easy subject for a consultation.

A few days later our doctor received a letter which he read over with Pat. On the physical side we were assured there was no steatorrhoea (thank God! it sounds awful, whatever it is) nor any other internal problem for us to worry about. He had just had something wrong with his digestion for a few days, that was all. But he offered his opinion that John's development needed some attention. While it was perfectly possible for him to be 'late-normal', a non-speaking three-year-old who seemed to have difficulty in understanding, let alone speaking; who had poor co-ordination, and who had elusive looks that sped away from your gaze, this was someone who needed an objective appraisal. The consultant stressed that he was making allowances for the fact that John had been kept too long in the waiting-room and was disturbed at the time. Possibly he was different at home—possibly not. . . .

'Well, what do you think?' asked our doctor. 'He looks O.K. to me. But do you want to take him to a child psychiatrist?' Mercifully he is the sort of doctor who believes in talking straight.

'Yes! I mean—we've got to know . . .' Pat replied.

'He might not be able to tell straight away,' cautioned the doctor.

Given that we'd been wondering more and more about John, it may seem odd that we were a bit shaken by the consultant's comments. But getting a direct comment from outside was very unusual.

'How can he judge when the poor kid was tired and screaming with boredom?' Pat asked me.

'It's a pity he can't see him at home,' I said. 'Then he might have a better idea of what John can do.'

But what exactly would the consultant decide if he could

see John at home? He would see how nice John could be; that he was really well behaved; that he knew how to fit in with what was asked of him, even if he couldn't answer a question or say what he was doing. The consultant would see him playing with Louise, listening to music, and he could hear him recite. . . . But what conclusions would he draw? I started to imagine him in the house, noticing things, comparing reactions, making up his mind.

Some seven years previously, at university, I had studied psychology. This meant, for the most part, knowing what a monkey's brain was like, and how rats learned their way round mazes. A small portion of the course, however, was called psychopathology, and so we were given a brief introduction to mental illness. I now searched in my old textbooks for some insight into what might be wrong with John—if anything. They weren't much help. My old lecture notes gave me a jolt as I discovered again the standards that average children are supposed to reach at different ages. There were also some comments about childhood handicaps and disorders. Nothing here made me think of John. All the syndromes sounded far more serious than anything we had seen in our own home. As for 'Kanner's Syndrome (autism)', all I had put down was:

> 'Psychotic alienation—kids ignore people—look through you—bang heads against walls—new, little known—happens with over-demanding parents, esp. teachers.'

I dismissed this too. John by no means ignored us, and he certainly never banged his head against a wall. Whenever I broke off from these fruitless researches I felt irritated. I decided I was fussing about for a dramatic cause when all John had was a development problem. He would be all right in the end.

I discussed my reading with Pat, and one night she surprised me with this question, 'Peter, do you think John is autistic?'

It was not long after we'd heard the consultant's comments. I said 'No' automatically.

'Well, what *do* you think is wrong with him then?' It was late at night. It had not been an easy day, and she was now crying.

'I don't know.' I made an effort to think and went on, 'Autism is far, far worse than what John's like—as far as I can remember. An autistic child has his own world, and doesn't know anything about ours at all.' The more I thought about it the more convinced I was. 'He's late. He's normal, but he's late. There are lots of things he's clever at, and he'll catch up on everything else in the end.'

This time Pat was not to be reassured so lightly. 'But can't we *do* something to help him catch up?' she demanded.

The only way, in fact, to stop being worried and depressed was to start doing things.

A friend of ours had heard of a book by Glenn Doman called *Teach Your Baby To Read*. As it was outlined to Pat a practical thought took shape in her mind: if John could be taught to read a few words it would get him used to saying things. We could then encourage him to say these words at the right moment, in the right situation. Once he realized how useful conversation was he would learn more phrases, and say them.

In those days we felt that there was some key to be found, some door that had to be opened. Then John would have everything at his mercy and all would be well. It was an encouraging belief, and in itself this did some good. But it was also cruel, because whenever John made some progress we felt instinctively that now, this time, we were at last almost there. And of course we weren't.

Glenn Doman's book was very heartening. To his specifications Pat made two large pieces of white card, one with 'Mummy', one with 'Daddy', in thick red printed letters that were five inches high. These she showed to John, saying the appropriate word loud and clear. He thought it was unusual, and fun. He repeated the words after Pat. The second time she showed one card and asked, 'What's this, John?' There was no answer, so she quickly said what the word was. He repeated it. They had one three-minute lesson every day after lunch. On the third day, as soon as he had finished his pudding, John went to the shelf where the cards were lying. He looked round expectantly. It now had the status of a ritual. Pat could miss out a lesson only at her peril.

The third day Pat showed the 'Mummy' card, and he said 'Mummy' before she could herself. She showed the 'Daddy' card—but he said 'Mummy' to that as well. Checking a sigh, Pat shook her head and said the right word. When he repeated it this time she said, 'Jolly good, John! Super! You've got it!' and he glowed with pleasure.

On the fourth day he got both cards right. From that point on he learnt about two new cards a day. These were mostly things that you can demonstrate easily—'Hand', 'Leg', 'Mouth', and so on. Whenever any of these words were introduced for the first time Pat pointed to the right part of his body. He soon copied her in this. She illustrated all words that came into the repertoire, pointing to herself for 'Mummy', to a picture of a tiger for 'Tiger', and so on. When the word 'Cat' was first used our new black cat Job was picked up and placed in front of him.

It all went very well for three main reasons. Having very short lessons meant that he was still eager to go on when he stopped. This meant that he wanted to pay attention the next day. Repeating the lessons day after day, as a ritual, made him happy with them. Finally Pat took very much to heart what Glenn Doman advises by way of reward. He was *never* told off or sharply corrected if he got something wrong. It was just ignored. If he did well one day he was praised as if he had done very well: if he did unusually well he was given to understand that he was no end of a scholar. This kind of ecstatic approval of what he had achieved absolutely delighted him. He lapped it up and sometimes even anticipated it. When he could see that the last card in a series was being presented to him, he said, 'Ta-ble. That's a table! Very, very good!' He clapped his hands, grinning, and began a little dance of triumph with Pat.

Very soon there were a lot of words that he could read—or perhaps one should say 'recognize'. And he had a pretty good idea of what to touch when he said things like 'Hair', 'Mouth' and 'Foot'. The size of card was reduced. Pat brought in some simple verbs, like 'Crying' and 'Going'. Soon she was able to string together several words for him, like 'Mummy is crying' or 'Job is running in the garden'.

At the beginning this was to be a session for John and John alone. Louise got plenty of attention. This was John's special time. Just after lunch Louise often had a rest, so it was a good moment. But one afternoon this was dramatically changed.

We had two rooms separated by bookshelves, open on both sides. Pat was going through John's cards in one room when she heard a voice interrupting. 'Dog!' shouted Louise, peering across one of the shelves and pointing determinedly at the particular card Pat had just raised up. She had got the right word in first, before John.

From that day on Pat held a joint session for both of them, and a separate session for John when she had the time. Louise was only just two years old. But she caught and overtook John in about a month. Soon she was actually seizing the cards from their shelf, and taking John through them. He seemed to enjoy sessions with her, about as much as with Pat. She was perhaps more sparing in her praise, but now and then she clapped her hands and congratulated her brother effusively.

By the time John was four he had about fifty or sixty words that he would read correctly most of the time. He took sentences in his stride, but he gave equal stress to each word. He wasn't reading statements so much as words that happened to be on the same line. Eventually he got the idea that the last word usually has to be spoken with a special intonation. But he was *imitating* that too, even when we were convinced that he was reading lines so naturally that they had to mean something to him.

The next area of effort was trying to narrow the gap that we could see widening between him and other children. Play groups I have mentioned. This was only once a week, so that Pat and a friend decided to hold a sort of dancing-class in our sitting-room once a week as well. Five or six children usually came, mostly three- or four-year-olds. Maureen, who had been an infants school teacher, led the singing games and the 'dancing' while Pat played the piano.

Having other children in his home seemed at first to be no different for John than if he met them at another house or the parish hall. That is to say he ignored them. This he did when they picked up his toys, played with them or broke them. He even kept away from Louise at these times—as if her enthusiasm for playing with others was a way of separating the two of them. But he got used to the fact that on certain days the lower part of the house was thrown open to a small number of children, whose names and faces became gradually familiar. They did certain things every week, sometimes singing, sometimes dancing, sometimes both at once. It became an accepted part of his world more quickly than play groups, which were on a larger scale, on foreign territory.

Moreover Louise was there to give him encouragement. Although she chose her partners mainly according to which of them she happened to be keen on that week, she often found time when the dancing began to give John a pull, and get him involved as well. When they formed a line to 'pull out the farmer's turnip', she could sometimes persuade him to grasp another child round the middle and pull in the right direction.

He got a certain amount out of this—not so much from the music or the dancing as from beginning to understand that playing with others can actually be fun.

For example, one singing game starts with one child holding his arms in front of him, with his hands together, like an elephant's trunk. He walks round the room, singing:

'One little elephant, balancing,
Balancing on a piece of string. . . .'

He is joined by other elephants, one verse to each new recruit. In the end the string breaks and they all fall on the floor. The idea of imitating elephants never entered John's head. Even now, pretending to be something else is a very difficult concept for him. The joke about elephants balancing on string, likewise, meant nothing. The tune never appealed to him much, judging from the fact that he never repeated it on his own, which he usually did with any tune that caught his fancy. He could be persuaded to follow the other children through the game—for a while. He soon forgot to keep holding his arms out, even if he remembered to keep behind the elephant in front. He didn't see the point of trying to walk like an elephant, and no doubt could not understand the instruction to do so. But he always loved the final scene where everyone fell down in a heap. This was fun. It meant something. One laugh a bit louder than the others used to be heard from the mass of threshing legs, trunks and bodies on the floor.

What this and other games showed him was that he did not need to be alone or with Louise to enjoy himself. It was also quite possible, even if he couldn't make out one word in ten of what they were talking about, to get some pleasure out of being with a gang of children. He needed to be convinced of this, and do-it-yourself dancing classes took him a certain way towards it.

A lot of John's contemporaries went to kindergarten—that is to a small private nursery school not far from us. The first time Pat thought about John going there it seemed too much of a challenge. Wouldn't it be better if he had a few more words in his armoury before trying his luck? We talked it over, and decided it was a kind of vicious circle. To learn to use language he might need to be with children his own age; before he had enough language with which to fend for himself it didn't seem fair to pitch him into the ring.

The mistress in charge was sympathetic, and suggested he might attend on two half-days a week. So he took his place in the school run for Mondays and Wednesdays. Pat waited for the mistress to comment on the result.

It was a relief to be told that, really, John 'was no trouble at all, and seemed to fit in quite well'. What actually happened is difficult to guess at, but it seems likely that he was much less trouble than he should have been if he had really been 'fitting in'. He was encouraged to join in things, but preferred to remain in a corner. Singing he would do with the others for a while. When they watched a children's television programme he ignored it. Dancing and games he avoided. Often no doubt he appeared to be listening to stories because he was well behaved and said nothing. We noticed that, unlike the other children, John never had any pictures or models to bring home with him.

But, with the benefit of hindsight, it was far better that he should have been accepted in the kindergarten than that he should have had to play around at home. What he constantly needed was to spend more time with more normal children. Almost any way of exposing him to them was better than nothing.

Chapter Seven

At long last we got an appointment to take John to see a well-known psychiatrist who is the consultant at G hospital. Because of a confusion of times and places Pat found herself yet again coping with a howling child. She had already been waiting for an hour at G when she was informed that the consultant had gone to his private address by mistake. She found a taxi and went on there, feeling not a little aggressive towards the hospital, psychiatrists and the world in general.

'How on earth do you expect to tell what's wrong with him when he's worn out, hungry and thirsty, and climbing up the wall with boredom?' She was surprised at the strength of her own voice when she put this to the consultant.

He was disarmingly kind, and himself helped make up some orange squash for John. But nothing could be done to put John into an agreeable frame of mind. He gurned, he screamed, he thrashed about. He ate a biscuit, but choked on it since he was trying to sob at the same time.

The consultant soon stopped trying to get answers from John. He glanced at him out of the corner of his eye from time to time while he asked Pat all about him.

One question stumped her: did John go upstairs putting alternate feet on each step, or did he put both feet on the same step before going any farther? Pat didn't know. It seemed to be rather important to the consultant.

Later, at home, we watched John on the stairs to see exactly what he did do. In fact he did put down both feet on each step before going on to the next. We had thought he was 'cautious', and so we hadn't noticed this. We had thought he was slow at reaching other children's standards for running, jumping and so on—possibly because he was a bit lazy. Now we wondered whether there was something seriously wrong with his co-ordination that was holding him back in all these things.

That afternoon the consultant told Pat, 'Well, he's certainly a late developer. He *might* have something more basically wrong with him, but at three and a half it's very difficult to be sure. It's quite possible that he'll develop normally, given time.' In the meantime he advised us to get John's sight tested as he thought that the way he looked at things was a bit odd.

His parting shot was interesting. 'Who was it, in fact, who wrote this letter about John to your doctor?'

'Dr M, at——'

'Not Dr M at A hospital?'

'Yes.'

'But he's the best child psychiatrist in the south of England. Why did you come to me?'

So we had an open verdict—or perhaps one should say, 'not proven'.

I noticed that Pat's attitude was changing. Before, we had talked, and argued, and had moods when we were anxious, followed by moods when we felt that everything was going to be all right. We were happy. Now Pat was difficult to cheer up. She was nervous when she spoke about John with other people. There were few times now when she said to me as I came back from work, 'John *has* had a good day today! Do you know what he did. . . . ?'

Our doctor prescribed iron for her; she found it hard to

accept any ideas I had for doing anything out of the ordinary at week-ends. It was winter now. She said it seemed to take all her strength to get through the week, let alone contemplate anything new on Saturday. At the same time she worried that John wasn't getting enough attention because of Louise, and that Louise was getting neglected because of John. Because of both of them, and because she didn't feel strong, she felt not enough was being done for *either* of them.

I can't remember how often I told her that there was a limit to what she could take on; that reading lessons, music sessions and dancing classes were far more than the average child got by way of special attention, to say nothing about games in the garden or walks across the common. But I was arguing against the symptoms and ignoring the cause of the trouble.

Inside me I knew what it was that we had to find out before we could enjoy peace of mind again. But I couldn't talk about it much. Apart from a stubborn feeling that John was simply 'a late normal' I had a twinge of disloyalty whenever I found myself wondering if John was mentally handicapped. It was letting him down, somehow, not to have complete confidence in him.

Saying we would just have to wait, and then we would know, was a facile and infuriating thing to say. But I said it. The more I said it, I told myself, the quicker Pat might realize fully that waiting was inevitable and get used to it.

But instead she got more nervous and looked more ill. Louise got on her temper, I got on her temper and so did John. It was worst when John did, because she felt instant remorse when she was angry with him. Once or twice she ran upstairs to our room and closed the door in order to avoid getting angry with the children.

Cooking was a double chore for Pat now because she

could no longer enjoy food without thinking about how she would feel afterwards. Every few days she complained of stomach pain, and nothing the doctor gave her seemed to send it away for long.

We quarrelled over odd things in those days. I was more nervy myself, I don't doubt, although temperamentally I show it less. Once I told Pat rather loudly to stop worrying about John because everything would be all right. He was like a plant, I said, that comes under suspicion in the greenhouse. Unearth it and examine the roots by all means—but at long intervals. Always lifting it out of the ground and studying it would not do it, or the gardener, the least bit of good.

'Just get it into your mind,' Pat answered me, 'that John is not a plant. He is a little boy. If you didn't hide yourself away in the garden so much you'd realize . . .'

I defended myself, I can't remember how. It was true about the gardening though. At week-ends it *was* easier to leave the family to grow by itself and attack the bindweed round the roses.

Pat wondered what we had managed to achieve with the reading, the music, the kindergarten and the dancing classes. How far was Louise, how far were the other children, drawing John into their world? Quite a lot was a fair answer. But it obviously wasn't enough.

John had learnt words, but not how to use them. He didn't seem to want to make conversation, and it was much harder now to imagine that this stage was just around the corner. He cried and lost his temper when he couldn't express what he wanted. Speech seemed as long a way off as ever, despite all. The gap between him and the others yawned.

In February, a low time of year in the best of years, Pat suddenly went to see our doctor again. She told him that she had to have another appointment with a psychiatrist for John or she would go crazy. I was all for waiting until after his fourth birthday, or a bit beyond—until a year after the appointment at G hospital. I was overruled, and now I am glad of it. It would have been utterly wrong to have gone on waiting further. The change in Pat afterwards entirely justified it.

Because of his reputation at G hospital, and no doubt also because he was nearer, Pat and the doctor agreed that John should see the A hospital consultant again. This time it was very different from the inquiry into John's digestive processes. This was the diagnosis that had started long before as a shadow in the corner of our minds, had grown despite all our attempts to deny its presence, and was now to be confirmed as a reality.

I have already described the scene in the little bedroom at the hospital where the consultant gave Pat his conclusions while John slept in the corner. That same evening I visited the hospital myself, as soon as I could get there from the office.

Pat was very composed when I saw her. She grinned to me as she put a finger to her lips, warning me not to wake John. A small bedside lamp was on. There were a few noises of trolleys and footsteps from the wards and corridors in the distance. This was just the hospital ticking over. It was a peaceful retreat from the cold, blustery wind outside. It seemed happy. I was quite sure that the consultant could not have made up his mind yet.

'Any idea when they're going to say anything?' I asked.

'What do you mean?'

'Well—you know. What they think about John.'

'He was in here about an hour ago,' Pat told me.

I knew who 'he' must be. I got up from where I was sitting, and then I wasn't sure what to do. It seemed colder than when I'd first come in. 'What did he say?'

'Sit down and break off some of that chocolate you've brought,' Pat advised me.

Knowing that she would be hating the hospital food, I'd brought a half-pound bar.

'Come on. And take some yourself.' Without changing breath she continued. 'He says John is definitely autistic. *Mildly* autistic. But he's quite definite about it.'

'Oh, God.' I slumped back in my chair and found I could not stop my hands from moving—rubbing against each other, clenching and unclenching.

'But we've expected it really, haven't we?'

'I suppose so.' I felt completely drained, and wondered why Pat gave no sign of feeling the same.

The consultant had strongly recommended that we should get hold of a book called *Autistic Children*, by Lorna Wing. I bought it next day, by which time Pat and John had come out of hospital. Each of us read it at one sitting.

All sorts of things fell into place. Endless crying for no apparent reason; unnaturally quiet behaviour as a toddler; beautiful features; the eye movements away from your face; speech difficulty; even the precocious musical interest, and the learning of long poems—all these things were mentioned in the book as being commonly found among autistic children. If we had had any doubts about what the consultant had told us this book would have settled them.

At the same time there were some things that had, mercifully, been spared us. We had never, for example, found John taking violent exception to the colour of new curtains and tearing them down. We had lost a certain amount of sleep—but some autistic children, apparently, need only a brief catnap around two in the morning and require attention for the rest of the night. Nor had our son gone in for head-banging; he had not refused all solid food; he had not set his mind against lavatories. Had he been like that, of course, we would have known sooner, but as it is we can only admire from a distance the courage of parents who have brought up severely affected children.

We couldn't wait for our next visit to the consultant. This was for the whole family. The weather warmed up in early March that year, and it was a more optimistic time to go. As we got into the car with the children I remember we were very cheerful.

Then, just before we reached the hospital, we ran into a squally shower. The windows misted as I had to edge into a narrow parking space in a street I didn't know. Suddenly Pat and I were arguing sharply about whether I would manage it, whether we ought to wait until the rain stopped, whether we would be late. All our nervousness broke out at once. Determinedly we mended our quarrel and walked out into the brisk winds that were rolling the clouds back.

This time the consultant glanced at Louise as much as he did at John. It was obvious he wanted a good look at her too. She wasn't all that easy to watch. First she discovered a toy-box under a bed, which she turned out on the floor in a matter of seconds. He spoke to her, and she grinned mischievously at him before diving into another box. This one contained medical instruments. As he sighed he smiled. She had made a good impression.

He had plenty of time for John too. But his attention was distracted by two parents who wanted to pump him as hard as they could, trying to understand all the problems about autism in thirty minutes flat.

'How far will he go?' Pat demanded at one point. It was the same question, more or less, that she had asked when she last saw the consultant. But we had to get back to it. She tried putting it a different way. 'When he's grown up, I mean. What are autistic *adults* like, exactly?'

'They must have existed of course—and they do exist. But it's been recognized such a short time ago that there simply isn't much evidence about what autism looks like in adults. There have been some cases, I believe, where the child gets better and better at understanding the world, and learning to live in it, so that he passes into it more or less normally. But most of them seem to need some sort of help.'

'Do you think John could be like that?' I asked immediately.

He took his time answering. 'It's hard to tell. People know more about it now, so he stands a better chance than he would have done in the past. And there's something about him'—he was regarding John carefully as he sorted through some of the toys on the floor with Louise—'there's something about him that suggests he might struggle his way through.'

These words gave me a very distinct flush of pride. He was not just autistic, he was John. He would struggle his way through—whatever that might mean.

'Is there a particular school we ought to be thinking about?' Pat wanted to know.

'Well——' He stopped, and seemed not to want to go on. A long time later we were to remember his pause and understand it. 'He ought to have some kind of special schooling, really. You see, if he's in an ordinary school he won't understand very easily what the teacher's saying, and she won't have time to stop for him. Maybe in the end—when he's talking, that is, and answering questions, and when he doesn't mind a lot of other children milling round him—then he might go to a normal school.'

He stressed that we shouldn't expect too much by way of scholastic achievement—ever. But he also pointed out that autistic children often had curious 'islands' of intelligence.

With some it was mathematics, some music, some art. Finding these islands made them happy. It provided a sense of purpose, and of pride. 'But for a start, he's got to learn to get along well with a lot of other children.'

'In the end,' Pat persisted, 'what will people think of him? Will he seem normal, I mean?'

'He'll probably always seem a little bit odd. But then, lots of people are like that.'

'And do you think he'll ever get married?' Pat went on.

'Hm.' He smiled at us as though to say he should have known that question was coming. 'That's the ultimate measure of getting on well with people, isn't it? Well, do you know . . . I don't think he will. . . . .'

I changed the subject quickly. 'What about this special schooling? What sort of thing do you mean? Is there a place near here?'

How naïve we were then!

'There's quite a good little unit—about twelve to sixteen children—at GC. Could you get him there, do you think?'

To my surprise Pat said immediately, 'We'll manage. Have you got the address?'

I had calculated the distance quietly to myself. If the roads were average for morning traffic it would take us about an hour to drive him there in the morning and an hour to get him back. 'Is there anywhere a bit nearer?'

'Of course you cut across the county boundary to get to this hospital,' the consultant went on, tackling the problem in his own way. 'You ought really to go to H, I suppose, to see what they have to offer. Would you consider sending him to a boarding-school?'

'Oh no!' Pat cried. Neither of us much likes the idea of boarding-schools for *any* children. I myself never went to one, and never wanted to, while Pat ran away from hers. For John, who showed such a strong need for routines, who clung to Pat or to me when in a strange place, it seemed utterly wrong.

The consultant was inclined to agree. But he advised us not to put it completely out of our minds for a later stage.

'Well, you had better see the Child Guidance Clinic at H. And contact the National Society for Autistic Children if you haven't done so already. They can give you a fair idea of how you stand on schooling locally.'

We had already telephoned the NSAC and applied to join. They sounded anxious to help, and supplied us with an assortment of titles of books and papers. One or two of these described operant conditioning—a specialized way of teaching in which correct reactions to stimulus words are reinforced by giving rewards. It was alarming to find that most of the important work in this area seemed to be taking place in New York, California, or in the Maudsley Hospital in South London: the teaching methods that experts seemed to think might be crucial for future progress were being developed by a few people, widely scattered.

The kind, but distinctly warning, voice at the telephone of the NSAC secretariat was also alarming. And a passage from Lorna Wing's book loomed larger in our minds. Towards the end she reviews services available for autistic children, and concludes:

> The parent of an autistic child must be prepared to make a great deal of effort on his own. He must pursue enquiries, write innumerable letters, and suffer long delays. . . .

We looked forward to the appointment at H with a certain foreboding now.

This contributed to a sudden change in Pat's mood. At the diagnosis itself she felt more relieved and determined than sad, while I was, for a while, completely dejected. As

I began to come up from under Pat began to get depressed. She now had a compulsion to scrutinize photographs of John as a baby for signs and symptoms.

The pride we had taken in him at the hospital where he was born—how simple and innocent that now seemed. Looking back, it was ironic that we accepted at face value the nurses' compliments on how handsome he was: this or 'regular features' we now knew could be expected in autistic children. At that hospital perhaps at that time something happened, or something started, that had meant he would be autistic. She looked back at one of the nicest and most important parts of her life in the sudden realization that at the core of it something was misleading, and wrong. Parents' and friends' comments, particularly the compliments, that lingered in the mind—all of them now had a slightly sinister tone. How much more had they suspected than they dared murmur to us?

The mood lasted for a few weeks, until she felt she could accept the dark side of these memories.

One question we had to come to terms with was this: how far had we ourselves, by denying John affection, and by imposing unattainable standards of behaviour and progress on him, actually induced, or helped induce, autism in him? This is the theory, in brief, of the 'refrigerator parents'. It's impossible to deny it by saying, 'Well, at least *we* weren't like that,' because if we were we would be the last people to know. Nor is it the kind of question that can be put to friends and relations, because the answer is obvious in advance. Nobody wants to admit that they are friendly with, or related to, 'refrigerators'.

The NSAC books and papers by and large denied that autism is an emotional disorder, stressing that all problems in autistic children can be logically traced back to a breakdown in communication. If some children have something wrong with their perception system, so that they cannot disentangle sounds, or things that they see, in the normal way; if, then, they have difficulty in combining, or drawing conclusions from what they hear and look at; and if they cannot easily reproduce sounds that would convey the meanings they intend; starting from this standpoint, it is quite reasonable to suppose that emotional problems creep in simply because the children get frightened of what they can't understand, or frustrated because they can't do or say much about it. The fact that some deaf and blind children develop autistic symptoms seemed to us to add a lot of weight to this view.

But we couldn't stop ourselves from looking back over the four years, and wondering if there wasn't some critical point, or some critical mistake, that might have started or increased the damage.

A strange coincidence made things easier for us. Although autistic children come at a rate of 1 to every 4,000 or so, for some reason the small firm at which I had first worked included another parent of an autistic child. (Later, I discovered, there was even a third, and we had all been contemporaries.) We made contact again through the society. He said, without bitterness, 'Don't for God's sake do what we did. For two and a half years we took Mark to a psychotherapist. It cost a fortune, and it did absolutely nothing for him.'

I have an open mind—I like to think—about psychotherapists. The categorical denial that anything at all had been achieved surprised me. 'Why did you go on for so long?' I asked him.

It wasn't easy for him to answer. 'When we started,' he said, 'nobody knew anything much about autism. They don't know much *now*, but at least they've got some idea about what to do to help them. We could not simply wait around for something to happen. It meant kicking ourselves every evening, wondering if the next day was going to be the same—the kiddie getting older, and nothing being done. So we began with a psychotherapist. She was persuasive, for a while . . . And later—we couldn't face the gap if we took Mark back from her.'

I asked my friend over, with his family. Their boy is a good deal older than John, and different in a number of ways. But the first impression he made was of being very like John in looks—a handsome, dark face; on the thin side, but strongly built. And his eyes wandered away from ours in a way we knew all too well. As soon as John saw him he went up to Mark and hugged him. John kissed him like a long-lost brother. Mark looked a bit embarrassed, but pleased. It was impossible not to think of John Wyndham's story, *The Midwych Cuckoos*, in which children with unusual eyes, and high but warped intelligence, are born to unsuspecting parents; as they grow up they recognize each other and prepare to take control of world affairs.

'How could *they* be refrigerators?' Pat asked me as we watched them leaving.

'They love Mark—and I can't imagine them ever having been any different. They're so easy-going I don't see how they could ever have demanded too much of a baby either.' I'd made my mind up about them, at least.

For a time we thought that some parents perhaps might have contributed, in some way, to their autistic children's condition. Others perhaps had not. But meeting a lot of parents through the NSAC made us realize that altogether there were none that we felt like putting in the first category. Some of them, whose children were particularly severe cases, had obviously been through hell—and it showed. These had learnt to make do with little sleep; and had retreated from social life as baby-sitters became less than keen to return to them, and as other families stopped asking them to 'bring along the children too'. They worried about schools; about ultimate hospitalization. But, meeting them properly, we saw that they were warm, friendly, and not so enclosed by their own troubles as to lose interest in other people's problems.

There was too big a gap between what these people seemed and what the psychotherapists suggested about them in the 'refrigerator parents' theory. We decided nothing—we simply stopped thinking about it.

Then we read a book by Bernard Rimland called *Infantile Autism*. He summarizes the case for looking for physical reasons for the fugitive mind, as opposed to assuming emotional breakdowns that hinder the brain from functioning normally. It has convinced us—but we still don't know *exactly* what causes autism, or even what autism is.

If autism were cut and dried, within fixed limits, there would be no room presumably for mildly affected children like John. Nor would there be any question about the best way to treat it, or the best teaching methods. At this time we were just on the point of finding out how big a question this is.

Chapter Eight

It was good news to hear at H that there was to be a new unit for autistic children set up at T, to serve the county. The psychiatrist Pat saw felt that this would be the obvious place for John to go to school. She did not question the diagnosis that had been given us a few weeks before.

Meanwhile we had heard about a special school in Ealing for autistic children. As it was supposed to be the only one specifically for them it seemed sensible to go and see it. They had a big waiting list we were told. John was young, we considered, and perhaps could wait longer than most. True, Ealing was far away, but if it was just right for him we might even move there.

We took John along for an interview, and were most impressed by Mrs Elgar who was in charge. John, in turn, impressed her and the consultant doctor—but too much. His reading, they said, showed that he was certainly capable of doing a lot. They would like to take him as he was very mildly affected, and would no doubt do very well with them. But there were other autistic children for whom Ealing would be more important. He might do as well in an ordinary school, provided it had small classes. In a sense it wasn't fair to take him.

So in the summer we made an appointment with the headmaster at T to go and see him with John. He was eager and friendly and showed us all around the school, which was basically for 'Educationally Sub-normal' children, but was to have this special unit attached. We were impressed with his new buildings and the equipment he had. There was also a happy atmosphere about the place.

The foundations of the building that was to house the unit were laid, and by picking our way across planks and blocks of cement we could see the shape it was taking. The headmaster explained the layout, and we were delighted with his enthusiasm. Even more impressive was the way he defined his role. He wanted to provide a stepping-stone, he told us, for children to use to get closer to their goal. If they reached a point at which they should leave and go on to a normal school, so much the better. That would be sufficient reward for his work.

We also met the unit teacher, J. She was to be one of two teachers looking after four children. She was a mother who had come back into teaching once her family had grown up. She admitted she had had no previous experience of teaching autistic children, but she had studied and thought about them a lot. She was determined to find out more. We liked the friendly way she made contact with John. Although he said nothing to her it was clear he felt positive towards her.

The headmaster remarked on the fact that John seemed very well behaved. This was a comparative reckoning, evidently, since John had in fact gone round the room picking up books and papers and murmuring to himself in a restless sort of way. It was implied that *some* children, on their first visit, had torn the place apart.

We were happy with the forecast that the unit would be ready by early September, so that John could make a start as soon as the autumn term began.

Meanwhile there was the summer. Encouraged by the approval we received at T, we continued with John's reading, and he progressed from large letters on cards to the

'Ladybird' reading series quite easily. This was a bit frustrating, however. With cards it was possible to get him to associate words with parts of the body, and simple but useful sentences (e.g., 'I want to go to the lavatory') with the appropriate direction. But books were quite different. He quickly learned to read easy books, like *We Have Fun*. He recognized words out of context—so it *was* actual reading. But he found it more convenient to apply his powerful memory to particular pages. This meant he didn't have to read the second time around. We tried to discuss with him what he had been reading. But whatever we said about the book he was on would set him off reading it to us again, parrot-fashion. It seems absurd, but it took ages to discover that although he could read *We Have Fun* perfectly, he had little idea of what 'we' meant; some, but a vague, idea of what 'have' meant; and absolutely no conception of what 'fun' could mean. He enjoyed what he read, in his own way. But, 'fun' . . . We couldn't show it to him, nor could he feel, taste or smell it. We pointed to a picture of children playing on a beach, and said, 'They're having *fun*, John.' Puzzled, he pointed to a beach ball and tried hopefully, 'That's a fun.'

Some words got through—ball, dog, water, shirt. . . . These he would repeat with particular delight. These words were practically the only ones with clear meanings. Colours too were all right for this reason.

That summer we went to a cottage by the sea in Wales. There was plenty of 'water', and he concluded that 'water' could be in the sea as well as in your bath. A simple step for Louise, but not so easy for John.

John gained a lot from that holiday—not least of all being the long hot days on the beach, exploring rock pools and shells. What he liked most, though, was to get into his trunks, walk into the sea up to his middle and wade solemnly through the water, staring down into it from time to time, and screwing up his eyes at the golden glints of sunlight on the surface of the ripples. Like so much else this became a ritual for him. He spent hours there, half immersed. 'Peter, for heaven's sake! He must be freezing out there.' I can hear Pat saying it now. I would agree, go down to the edge, throw the ball towards him and try to lure him into a game on dry land. He accepted the ball in the water, but protested loudly when he realized he was being lured out of his preferred element.

However much he liked the sea, he jibbed at the idea of floating or swimming. We tried holding him up, in the shallows, and tilting his body into a swimming position. But, as soon as he felt his head being lowered towards the water, he shouted and hung onto us, tight and grim. We soon lost any feeling that he could be jollied out of this, and we left him to paddle.

That summer we discovered in a newspaper article that there was such a thing as 'music therapy'. It suggested that all sorts of handicapped children could be encouraged to learn through music what they could not pick up naturally. As John enjoyed music so much it seemed an obvious thing to try with him.

Pat visited a music therapist, and was given a lot of ideas. 'We've got to buy some chime bars,' she murmured happily one evening.

'Chime bars?' I raised an eyebrow. Then, 'How much?'

'Not *too* much,' Pat assured me.

When she explained that each chime bar gives you a single, pure tone I was very surprised. 'Must be rather boring,' I thought privately. But John loved them. He had a session a day with Pat, taking each bar out of its little box, setting them up to form an octave and learning to play on them with a kind of drumstick.

'Hallo, D . . . Hallo, E . . .'

He learned to put down each bar opposite the right letters, which Pat drew in red on cards.

What he actually learned through music at this time is difficult to define. He certainly developed a sense of when to say 'hallo' and 'goodbye' to people (not just chime bars). And he greatly enjoyed it all.

Coming back, we looked forward to John's first term at school. There was no uniform to buy, and of course we could not discuss it with him. Nevertheless it was exciting in prospect, and we said to him 'You're going to school soon, John! That'll be fun!' every few days. We thought he might get used to the word 'school', if not the reality.

But school was a long time coming. Hearing nothing about the transport arrangements—we had been told that a car or a minibus would be collecting him, and other children, for the long journey to T and back—we rang up the school. Unfortunately, they told us, the building still wasn't finished. They were now hoping it might be ready by October.

His teacher, J., got in touch with us a few weeks later and said, 'I'm simply fed up with waiting. *Nothing* is being done. The builders haven't been near the place for ages. Do you think you could put some pressure on, or something?'

Pat picked up her pen with her right hand just as she was putting the phone down with her left. She wrote to two local newspapers, pointing out that autistic children, because of their handicap, have a lot of ground to make up. Learning to speak by the time they are seven is considered crucial to their whole development. Surely it was heartless to down tools, waste precious time and spoil their best chance of getting on terms with life.

One newspaper made it clear, when Pat followed through by telephone, that they had no interest in the story. It was difficult not to believe that they were unwilling to provoke the council, or a local business interest. The other paper, however, was new to the district. They phoned round, checking what Pat had told them, and ran a strong story. The very next morning builders returned to the site and finished everything in five days. In mid October a van called at our house in the morning to take John to school.

Pat went with him, the first day, so that she could help out if John suddenly became distressed by any of the bewildering things that would be done around him, and said to him. In fact, although everything was strange, he seemed quite content to make the journey, and to be delivered into J.'s hands. Pat left school early, and was very pleased when John was brought back by the van, calm and in good order.

A few weeks later Pat visited the unit. She was anxious to learn how John was settling down. There were then four children in the unit, including John. Two of these others were markedly more autistic than John and distinctly 'hyperactive'—relentlessly on the move, never stopping at anything for long. The fourth child was a special case by any standards. K. was hyperactive with a vengeance, and apt to be violent. He had no speech, understood little and was strong for a six-year-old. When Pat walked into the unit the first thing she saw was K. taking John by the hair and thumping him into the wall.

J. was in the process of losing a stone and a half in weight. She had a wonderful gift of giving herself, constantly and affectionately, to the business of getting the children to register her presence; to like her; to enjoy doing things with her; and, eventually, to concentrate on what she wanted to show them. She was making a lot of progress with John, and with two of the other children. But it was really unkind of fate to launch K. at her. The greater part of both teachers' nervous energy had to be devoted to watching and controlling him. Otherwise much of the school property and the lives of the other children were at risk.

Pat discovered that John was being very resilient to being thumped against the wall. He began to get used to the fact that the world is not full of people who will treat him nicely. It was unpleasant news sometimes, but he was learning to take avoiding action. On occasion he had to be rescued—and quickly too—but the experience must have had its good side as well.

What J. tried to do was to attach herself to John for long spells during the day, as far as she could. She believed that the more he became used to having her as a constant companion the more he would feel inclined to share experiences: he would stop existing just by himself, and he would communicate.

There was no formal teaching then. John and his teacher went from one piece of equipment to another, in the unit, and she saw to it that whatever he did they did jointly. They went hand-in-hand round the school itself, sitting in on any classes that seemed to interest him. Because J. kept up a running commentary, whatever each of them did, he was encouraged to feel that human beings get more fun out of what they're doing if they use words.

Obviously J. was limited in the extent to which she could carry out her programme. The other children deserved attention as well. Sometimes K. needed two teachers, using all their strength. Added to this restriction was the time problem: the children were at school only between the arrival of the bus and its departure in the afternoon, after lunch. If the traffic was bad it meant that a large proportion of school time was gone. All this made John's teacher's plan less easy to carry out.

John seemed rather indifferent about school. We couldn't

ask him anything about it. He never said anything or gave any sign when leaving home or coming back that he either enjoyed it or hated it. When she went there Pat could see he was happy enough, despite being pounced on by K. He was obviously very fond of his teacher, although he didn't talk much to her. But one point worried her.

'There was a little girl there,' Pat reported to me that evening. 'She keeps tearing up newspapers all the time. Don't you think it's a bit suspicious?'

I knew what was *really* worrying Pat, and it concerned me too. She didn't have to spell it out. John had started on newspapers too. But this was less alarming than the thought that John, who seemed less handicapped than the other children at the unit, might pick up all sorts of weird behaviour from them. The idea that he might copy some of K.'s habits was thoroughly awful.

'We can't tell, can we?' I went on after a bit. 'They'll move him into the main part of the school when he gets older. Specially if they see he's getting worse because of the others.'

'What if it's too late then?' Pat muttered.

In fact newspaper tearing stopped pretty quickly. John was using more words now, and sailing through the 'Ladybird' series in the evening. Louise, who shared his room, was well ahead in reading ability, but he was moving at a perfectly respectable pace, bearing in mind he was not yet five. 'Want a reading, please!' he announced, whenever he doubted that he would get his share as well as Louise.

Even more impressive was his new mastery of certain phrases, together with the right moment to bring them out. 'Thank you' and ''Scuse me, madam,' came into this category—although 'madam' was used without discrimination as to sex. But if he bumped into you he was obviously proud of knowing what to say.

Another good thing was that he was running better, and walking in a more alert way. We wondered how much K. had contributed to this! When John was still two we had bought him a small tricycle. Louise had learned to use it, but he had not. We bought him a larger one on his fourth birthday, thinking, 'Large boy—needs to learn on a large tricycle.' But Louise had practically taken that over too. Now with her help he could work the pedals by himself. He only did it downhill, or on the flat, but it was heartening. His arms got stronger, and now he could do 'wheelbarrows', if I held his legs, just as well as Louise.

How much all this was due to the good work at T school, we don't know. Having J. as his teacher, who worked very hard with him, must have contributed a lot.

But the journey to T became more variable as the spring term wore on. John came back looking distinctly tired. It was a long way to go for a child who had just turned five. It occurred to us that the older he got the more the actual journey would seem to be eating into his school day.

Then he caught mumps; as did Louise. He was ill only for a few days, but he was tired for a long time afterwards. Many of his phrases seemed to disappear. Much of his newly developed curiosity and his sense of fun vanished. An arduous journey seemed very wrong for him.

When summer arrived we took a close look at several schools. The prep school at which we had reserved him a place at eighteen months was fiercely competitive: it would have worried us, even if John had been normal. There were two other local private schools, both of which have a tradition for caring about children who do not fit easily elsewhere. One of them, we felt at the interview, might have been quite good for John. But they made it clear that they would accept him only if we agreed to send Louise as well. They were anxious, they explained, to avoid turning into a school that catered mainly for handicapped children. This seemed too much of a restriction on Louise, quite apart from the feeling of blackmail. The other of these two schools said, fine, yes, they would take John all right. But Pat was flabbergasted at how casual they were: they scarcely bothered to listen to what she had to say about him, or even to look at him. He would be another name on the books—fine. The building smelled heavily of damp; and the teacher in the kindergarten form had had no formal training at all.

There was still the local primary school. Pat got an introduction to the teacher of the youngest class and discussed John with her. The teacher was very intrigued. She explained that, running a class of thirty to forty children, she could scarcely give John any special attention. But she seemed game for a try.

The headmistress of this school was much less optimistic, although she agreed to her teacher's suggestion that John might attend for a day, for a trial run. This was possible because their term did not quite coincide with that of T. Pat took John along in the morning and introduced him. The teacher encouraged several children to say hallo to him, and make him feel at home. Pat went away with two fingers firmly crossed.

Lunch over, she walked around nervously, wondering how long to leave him before picking him up. When she arrived the teacher was all smiles. 'He's settled down fine,' she announced. 'No trouble at all.' He seemed to be liking it too. He protested when he was drawn away from the motorway flyover some children were constructing to get his coat on.

Two of his 'helpers' kept pace with him as Pat led him to the door.

'Please, miss, why can't he stay with us?' asked one.

'Maybe he will, sometime,' Pat told them. She had to tug John to the doorway, since he kept glancing back enviously at the motorway.

'Please,' asked the other one, 'what *country* does he come from?'

Pat looked at him in surprise.

'He doesn't seem to understand us,' the little boy explained.

'Oh, John's English all right, but he doesn't talk very well yet,' Pat said quickly.

Although the teacher declared that she was perfectly willing to take John, the headmistress would not let her. 'There will be a new headmaster taking over in a year's time,' she said to us. 'It would not be fair to commit him to taking your son before he has a chance to decide himself.'

Looking back, we are not at all sure it would have worked anyway; but it was very disappointing at the time.

John was back at school for the summer term now, and we had made no progress towards getting him an easier journey or integrating him with normal children. He still seemed rather jaded. Sometimes we felt this meant he ought to stay at T, where he would be sure of a slow, gradual introduction to any kind of school work. Sometimes it seemed that T, and the journey there and back, must be at fault, holding him back.

The end of term came, and we went to Wales again on holiday. Despite the facts that it rained a lot, that Louise had tonsillitis, that Pat was now at an uncomfortable stage of pregnancy, and that the girl who was to have helped us never appeared—it still seemed to do John a lot of good. The change, the easy pace, pottering round the farm that he may dimly have recognized, discovering the sea and the rocks again, all these things, with no help from ourselves, meant a great deal to him. He refused to swim, and refused to play with other children. But he ran, laughed and splashed, and was good company. When we drove back, it seemed absurd that we had nearly given up hope of finding normal schooling for him.

We got in touch with the psychiatric social worker at H, who promised to look for some school that might act as a suitable bridge for John, between the T unit and an ordinary class. Meanwhile he should stay where he was.

This conversation took place about three weeks before Pat was due to have the baby. Term began on the day immediately before the baby came. That morning we waited for the van to come and take John to school as it had always done. It didn't arrive. Pat phoned up the school about ten o'clock.

'Oh, don't you know?' the secretary said. 'John's not being picked up this term. We're sorry, but no transport beyond H can be arranged any more.'

I had a few days off work, so I was able to amuse John for part of that day. I rang everyone I could think of who might have the influence to help get him to school. In the end a splendid social worker who had entirely different responsibilities took it on himself to arrange for John to be picked up by a coach collecting mentally handicapped children for a training centre at H. He also arranged for the T van to pick up John from the centre. I told Pat that the new system had been confirmed at T just before she started labour.

The next day a large coach, with four or five mongol children aboard, plus a worried-looking boy with nervous hands, and an old lady to look after them all, pulled up at the front door. A large boy at the back gave me a great 'Hallo!' and waved vigorously once John had taken his place. We greeted each other regularly after that.

Unfortunately the double trip didn't help John all

that much. Because of the cut-down in transport services generally the T van had to take a very circuitous route, collecting more children than before. His teacher told us that his day had become one long bus ride, punctuated with an hour or two at school around lunch time. She was reduced to driving out of her way to H herself, when she could, in order to get him to school reasonably quickly and happily.

We rang the psychiatric social worker several times. The headmaster, we gathered, was very pleased with John's progress, and was making personal efforts to find him a school that would be 'absolutely right'. It was never possible to talk to the headmaster on the telephone.

In January J. rang me one evening to say that her unit was no longer to be just for autistic children. Other children, emotionally disturbed, maladjusted, schizophrenic possibly, were to be added to it. There was pressure from elsewhere in the school for the unit teachers to take on more pupils, in order to 'spread the load' more fairly. J. had held out for individual attention for autistic children at all costs, but a kind of compromise now seemed inevitable. She had rung us to explain why she thought this was bad from John's point of view: he needed all the attention he could get, just as he was beginning to react to a teacher as to a friend from whom he could learn things. Autistic children, she told us, were out of favour at the school anyway. They were getting rid of K. for a start. Nobody knew what would happen to him, but he wasn't wanted any more at T. John was counted a partial success for the unit, but this wasn't enough to save it in its present form. The headmaster wasn't anxious to have autistic children around now because the arrangements set up for them led to dissension among the staff.

'Well,' I said at last, 'it seems a shame. Obviously we've

got to go on looking for something better for John. How's he getting on this term, by the way?'

There was a pause at the end of the line. 'Oh,' she said. 'He hasn't been to school yet.'

I shouted 'What?' down the phone. For three mornings now John had been picked up by the coach in the morning and brought back by it in the evening. What had happened to him in between?

J. had turned up at T as usual, on the first day of term, to be told the roads were too icy for the school van to collect the autistic children. No one had told *us*.

I rang the friendly local social worker who did some detective work. The people at the centre in H had been surprised, at first, that no van came for John. Then they produced some toys for him and gave him lunch together with the severely handicapped children who were regularly there. He wasn't old enough for the woodwork or cooking classes and was left to his own devices. At going-home time he simply joined the coach with the others.

This had gone on for three days. All the snow had cleared. Our social worker rang up T to ask whether the van would be running again soon. Had he not done so—it's too easy, perhaps, to over-dramatize things in retrospect—but had he not done so, in a firm voice, it seems possible that John would have been simply forgotten.

Few things are so infuriating as the knowledge that your child has been shunted round (whether deliberately or not), and that because he couldn't describe it there was nothing you could do. It took me about a day to climb down from the ceiling. As for Pat, she was speechless. We had to find another school for John.

Yet we didn't take him away, for fear he would miss a lot of valuable time.

There are two points I want to make out of all this. I

hope they justify my going through this chequered period in detail.

First, no parent can afford to think for a moment that, whatever his or her child might be, the Education Authority —or *any* authority—will have everything organized for him. Authorities exist to do a good job for the majority, although they now have an obligation to provide education for all. The parent exists to make sure that his child actually benefits, actually gets a suitable opportunity for education. Countless times we were told, 'Oh, don't worry—it's going to be all right.' Whenever we hear the phrase again now it makes us shiver with apprehension. It's not going to be true unless you *make* it true.

With hindsight it's all pathetically logical. If you have an unusual child, a special case to put, you have to be able to discuss this with an individual. An organization tries to be greater than the sum total of the individuals within it. Therefore when an authority suspects that a special case is coming the individuals are liable to avoid having too much to do with it: they feel that, as individuals, they might get too much involved. That would be transgressing the code of their organization. Most of them, then, let special cases drift along in the hope that they will sort themselves out.

What a parent must do with a special problem is to establish early on *who* are the individuals with responsibility in the authority; *how* they can best be contacted, preferably person-to-person; *what* are the rules of the game they are playing, i.e. who has to protect whom in the organization, what are the official and unofficial policies that might be restricting individuals from taking individual action. Had we known this ourselves, at the beginning, we could have saved a lot of time and worry.

Secondly, a new building with marvellous equipment, all especially designed with autistic children in mind, by itself means absolutely nothing. For success you need good teachers with a lot of time and patience, and with people behind them who understand that dramatic improvements overnight are a rarity. A flexible system, allowing interchange between the unit and other classrooms, could help: other teachers might feel that they too were sharing in the education of the autistic children. Possibly units for autistic children with different levels of severity are also needed—but our experience is limited on this question. In any event, if John had not had J. his time at T would have been a dead loss.

Chapter Nine

I mentioned a new baby in the last chapter. This was the result of a conscious choice. Louise arrived before we knew what John was really like. But later we had to ask ourselves whether the pleasure that a larger family would bring outweighed the problems that might increase as John grew older. We decided that a larger family was right.

There were several obstacles in the way. The biggest was a third-month miscarriage, which laid Pat low for several weeks. Physically everything went all right after that. But there were two au pairs in succession who had to be asked to leave, and there was the tedious business of finding replacements. Next, the house we were living in was large enough to fit in another baby but not another growing child. We decided to ask an architect round to draw up plans for an extension.

By the time September came round, and Simon arrived on a bright sunny afternoon, it seemed only a just reward for Pat after all her hard work. This was in a downstairs room, and I was there with one of the best midwives ever. She was a splendid character, utterly professional but human as well, who knew all about the National Childbirth Trust methods. She radiated a sense of organization and confidence while remaining friendly. Simon proved harder going than Louise had been, having swelled to a full nine pounds. But, with pethalorfan to help, Pat kept in control throughout, and enjoyed the achievement of actually guiding the delivery herself. After five hours of it the midwife, Pat and I had developed a marvellous esprit de corps as a team. The doctor felt rather out of things when he arrived. He said, 'You seem to be doing all right then,' complimented us with a grin and continued on his round.

In the kitchen a short way away the children were having tea with a temporary nanny. I went in to them, and my smile told them most of what they wanted to know. John clearly understood that something important had happened without understanding what it was. Louise demanded, 'Can we see him? Can we see him?'

I took them in, and they all saw how happy Pat was, and what a large baby she had produced. Unlike Louise, he was not at all puffy and much more placid about being in the world.

I told John, 'This is baby Simon, John. Baby Simon.'

He smiled broadly at his brother, and poked tentatively at his shawl. 'Baby Si-a-mon,' he repeated. Simon remained 'Si-a-mon' for many months.

Louise was intoxicated with this motherhood business. The next morning, when I went into the sitting-room for the first time, I saw that all her soft animal toys had been placed in snug corners of the furniture, wrapped in nappies snatched from the airing cupboard. Even Job, who was curled up on a chair, had a nappy over him. (He is a cat who will sleep through anything.)

She also drew pictures of Simon, tightly swaddled, that made him look like a jumping bean. Finally she demanded to know when she could have a baby herself.

John was intrigued by Simon, though not nearly to the same extent. He smiled when he saw him. It's not easy to describe, but he showed he had a sense of something important and happy visiting the house.

'Did you ever actually think,' someone asked me at work,

'that possibly your next child might have been—er—handicapped too?'

After the event it was easy to reply that we had discounted any risk, and been proved right. But the possibility had certainly crossed our minds.

We had learnt from Rimland's book that families with an autistic child seldom include other cases of mental handicap, and very rarely include a second autistic child. But I have a feeling that we wanted a third child so badly that even if the risk factor had been as high as one in three, we would have had one. Partly, I suppose, we wanted to prove something—which may not be very laudable. But, basically, we wanted Simon.

All our relatives were pleased. At Simon's christening party it was interesting to observe them with John. They had grown used to the idea that to John you said something loudly and slowly with a smile; then you watched while he turned down your conversational opening; having done your duty you could pass on to someone else. I am not criticizing—it's not much fun forcing yourself to try to relate to a child you don't understand, who gives little encouragement. This time, though, they saw something different. They saw him well behaved in church; passing nuts round to people when asked to at the party afterwards; exchanging glances with people when they looked his way, or spoke to him; even saying some things in his turn.

In the kitchen a plate of canapés had been left, unwisely, on top of the fridge. Job was making his way towards it, from the window-sill, flashing his tail and wondering whether to attack the anchovies or the smoked salmon first. 'Down, Job! Get down, Job!' John cried before anyone else noticed, or found the right words to use. Swearing, our cat dropped to the floor and scuttled away. 'That's a naughty cat!' John added with a delighted smile.

And yet anyone who asked him a direct question such as 'How old are you?' or 'How do you like your school, John?' got no reply.

The children who came to the party got further with him, on the whole, than their parents. One of them led him by the arm and said things like 'Do you want some cake, John?' to which he answered 'D'you want some cake, please?'

Anyone who explored with him the territory he was getting to know could end up by extending that territory a little.

Anyone demanding 'What's your name?' would get an answer that we had taken care to teach him, along with his address and telephone number. He repeated the question 'What's your name?' adding 'My name is John Rowlands.'

How far his name had 'meaning' for him is a difficult question. It could have been no more than a sort of trigger-word: hearing 'your name', he replied 'John'. But it *was* more to him. If he looked at pictures he had not seen before he could point accurately at himself, asked or unasked, and say 'That's John.'

Most of the people who came to that party were agreeably surprised at John's advance. Yet he still gave them plenty to be puzzled about. He had grown fast, and was tall for his age. This taxed them when they tried to place him accurately in time. 'Let's see,' they said dubiously, anxious not to be tactless with us, 'he must be—how old now . . . ?'

It was all very gratifying on his good days. There were bad ones too. Each time we calculated how long John spent in the school bus we felt a gnawing sense of time slipping by, and our being incapable of doing much about it. The thought of him stuck there, just sitting still, looking out of the window—empty time relieved only by an occasional word from one of the mongol boys. What kind of education could this be?

Once at school the important thing for him had been his close link with his teacher. But now this seemed to be in danger. Short of winning the pools, and building our own school, the prospect was bleak. On John's bad days we sometimes demanded 'Just how did we get into this?'

We began to understand how some parents progressively ignore one of their children (who may be perfectly normal) and wrap themselves up entirely in the future of the others. It's not that they necessarily dislike the child; rather, they lapse gradually into lack of interest. I imagine their despairing of helping him to develop in what they feel is the best way. Instead, they resign themselves to the idea of the system (school, apprenticeship or whatever) taking control. Before, I couldn't understand them. But it's all too easy—particularly if the other children are bright, lively and competing for attention. I had a glimpse, then, of how easily we could have established a pattern of thinking about Louise and Simon, and gradually letting John drift further and further from our concern. If you know time is against you there is a limit to how long you can stand fighting it without making headway.

If John had just remained as he was for more than a few months, then perhaps we might have despised ourselves. If he had really seemed to be suspended in time, playing with the same things, making the same noises, we might have said to ourselves, 'That's his level then. Possibly a few more small improvements. But why kick ourselves because we can't see how to get him to talk, to receive education, to make friends with other children?'

But now and again he would surprise us. He would discover a new word; or he would rediscover an old one, this time using it more accurately. And his interest in music could still catch us unawares. One Saturday morning I went out to the garage to check over the car. As I peered under the bonnet I whistled a bit of Beethoven's Third Symphony to myself. I stopped and looked around for an oil-rag. As I found one I saw John's face peeping round the corner of the garage doorway. He slithered along the side of the car until he was with me, and said, 'Mm, mm. I want a—I want a—Please! I want a——' Then he hummed part of the theme back to me. 'I want a—(hum)—please!'

I completely forgot about checking the oil. John stared very closely at me, not at my eyes, but at my lips, and hummed with me as I whistled to him. He looked very solemn, and insistent. We went through it three times. Then he was satisfied. As he made his way back he paused and pointed to the car. 'That's a car,' I was told. 'That's a red car.' And he went.

When he was alert and friendly like this it was impossible not to hope that somehow, somewhere, we might find the right school for him—so that the years in which he *could* learn to adapt to the world would not just drift away.

We thought seriously about America sometimes, and the new methods of teaching autistic children, pioneered in California and in New York. If we sent him there, John might arrive on a tide of educational planning for children like him. He might get individual attention, plus the latest teaching developments at the University College of Los Angeles. If we saved, if I angled for a job . . .

Several things turned us against this idea. First, a perfectly good specialist school in this country had turned John down—because, to simplify, he was too like a normal child. This could also happen in New York or anywhere. Then there was the stream of news of rioting in American cities, of increasing tension and violence between black and white. We did not want to expose our young family to that.

Besides, we enjoy England too much to be able to leave it easily. But the final issue was the strange story told by an Australian couple we met about this time.

These people had two sons, the elder of whom was autistic. His condition was not understood in Australia, and he was not treated sympathetically beyond the circle of his immediate family. Father and mother decided they had to go abroad, to England, to get reasonable consideration and teaching for their son. Having covered half of the world to get here, they found themselves buying a house with a postal address in H county, but physically situated a hundred yards across the border, in the county of B. Having applied to the county unit for H, they saw it and decided they liked the look of it. Their boy was provisionally accepted—then turned down by certain authorities who observe the county boundaries meticulously. The Australians sighed, then asked the B authority, 'All right, then. What can you offer us in B?'

They were told that the only place in B suitable for their boy was full. Perhaps if they looked around they might find the right sort of private school . . . They ended up selling their new house at a loss, missing half a term and moving into the heart of H county.

This cannot just happen in England. Something like it could easily happen to us if we went to the States. It convinced us, irrationally perhaps, that we would do better to stay where we were. On our own territory at least we knew the lie of the land. This story also made us feel we ought to take a more active part in what the NSAC were doing, to help press for more schools for autistic children—not just for John.

It occurred to us that the brunt of John's education was falling more and more on Louise. One point made about brothers and sisters of autistic children in Lorna Wing's book is that these children tend to get saddled with more responsibility; gradually this puts their childhood out of balance and they acquire 'a maturity out of keeping with their years'.

We have tried to help her in various ways. We chose a school for her which, although a day school, will hopefully supply her with a separate and secure world. This school appealed to us as a happy place, which takes girls at five and sees them right through their school life. She could have friends, then, in the same form, for ten years or more. It was also conveniently placed, in case we found ourselves having to move to a nearby county for John's sake. And, if the worst came to the worst, Louise could always board there, either for a short or a long period. Here, we hope, she need not feel weighted down with obligations.

In the same spirit, we have tried to establish equal partnership between John and Louise in everything. They both get asked to put their toys away—even if it sometimes means placing a toy in John's hands and pointing to the toy-box. Equalizing their treats has been, and still is, considerably more difficult. Louise would watch a Punch and Judy show quite happily, while John would fidget because he didn't get the point of what was going on, or why the other children were laughing. To deprive Louise of the chance to enjoy this kind of thing seemed unfair; but it might be unfair on others to put John where he would suddenly bound up, walk round and block people's view. We had to try to choose treats for both of them that were 'safe bets', as well as attractive.

They both had to take the blame for mischief too. Although it is Louise who always answers, if we hear crashing glass we have always tried to shout, 'John and Louise! What on earth's that?' followed by 'Which of you was it?' and, if appropriate, 'You naughty children!'

At music sessions each was given a turn with the same instruments, even if it meant 'guiding' John into making a choice sometimes. In the garden, if one was issued with a trowel the other would get a hand-fork. If Louise asked for some wallflower seeds to plant, John would be given some aster seeds. Each would get the same size flower-pot, with little stakes marked 'Louise's flowers' or 'John's flowers'. He has never seemed to connect the green shoots in the pot with the seeds he pressed into the soil two weeks before, but he has always liked having his own flower-pot when Louise has had hers. This indicates to *both* of them they are essentially equal partners.

All this organized equality has meant taking more time. Often, obviously, we simply haven't had the patience to continue with it. During this period in his life, when John seemed virtually to be living on school buses, patience was at a premium. It was so much easier to say, 'Louise, for God's sake, clear all this junk out of the sitting-room, and get John to help you.' She did it all right, but it gave us a nagging feeling that we were setting up an imbalance between them that would do neither any good in the end.

While in the garden, insisting that it was now John's turn to go on the swing became a deadly chore. Louise would get the message from us that she ought to share the swing with her brother, rather than hogging it, and persuading him to give her a push every now and then. She got into the habit of observing the letter of the law; getting off, then saying (rather too loudly), 'Now, John, up you get! It's your turn on the swing!' John, smiling, would get on the seat. He would be pushed for a few seconds. Finally (less loudly this time), Louise would say, 'Off you get, John—it's my turn now,' easing him off again. She could then install herself for a good five minutes or so.

A lot of the time our campaign for fair shares just didn't seem to make any more sense. He took to objecting strongly at being led into garden games with other children when they came to visit. Sometimes we managed to start them off playing together—running races, or playing follow-my-leader, or making roads for toy cars in the sand-pit. After a while I would look up from my gardening and not be able to see John at all. Worried, I would check the side gates, although he has never shown any interest in going away by himself. Passing inside the house I would find him, curled up on the sofa. Once I caught myself saying, as I saw him there, 'If only he were asleep'—that is, not just staring at nothing.

Sometimes it was difficult to see how he could ever make any more progress. There was a difference, surely, between his not being able to do things and not wanting to do anything. We could help him compensate for the first but not for the second. Other children seemed to be so much more *alive*. They made up games, they competed with each other, they imitated us, they made us feel they were really in love with life. John, somehow, existed. He was among us, but as if by accident.

Even if they came on his worst days, however, my parents and Pat's mother never betrayed any wavering in their confidence. Pat's mother clearly felt that, so long as he greeted her with a kiss when she arrived, there couldn't be much that would stop him. My father was more actively admiring. He liked to observe John from a distance, and point out little ways in which he was catching up.

Pat and I were a bit suspicious of indulgent grandparents' talk. But we were both struck by one very perceptive comment that my father made during this period. He had noticed once how John had hovered near, but not too near, a group of visitors. Suddenly John had jogged up to them, and said, 'Hallo, John!' When our visitors turned, smiled and repeated encouragingly, 'Oh, hallo, John!' he was off down the garden again. 'Sometimes,' my father decided, 'you can see him coming through the forest, right up to the edge of the clearing—he looks in, for a moment, and then he's away.'

But how could we get him to stay?

One Sunday afternoon when we were feeling particularly low John gave us a hint that he might be able to surprise us in the end. Louise, who now read anything she could get hold of, had enjoyed a story about some older children (of the age that was *supposed* to be reading the book). They had climbed a big tree to signal for help. What could be more fun than to try to scale our walnut tree? It was, after all, far enough down the garden for parents to be unlikely to object.

Suddenly, from the garden depths, we heard a shout of triumph—first from John, then from Louise. We went down to investigate and couldn't see them at first. High up in the branches they looked rather small. Louise, in fact, was only half way up, but very satisfied with her success. John had gone higher, attempting branches that were too alarmingly distant for his sister. His grin of pleasure radiated down to us from the tree-top like a Cheshire cat's.

We were naturally worried at finding we had arboreal children who liked climbing dangerously high. But it was wonderful to see John all at once daring something, like any ordinary mischievous boy. In a discouraging winter it seemed a good harbinger of what might yet come.

Chapter Ten

One afternoon Pat had a telephone call from the school. John wasn't very well—could she come over and collect him? She left Louise and Simon with a neighbour and set off.

At T she was relieved to find that it was nothing worse than that he had been sick. He still looked green, and quite obviously couldn't take the long bus journey back.

'He'll be ever so glad he's going home by car—won't you, Johnnie?' J. said as she helped him into his coat.

'Doesn't he like the bus at all then?' Pat asked her.

'He's taken right against it. It's all we can do to get him in sometimes.'

Pat bit her lip. She drove back slowly and as smoothly as possible, glancing at John in the mirror from time to time. One of the compensations (so we had hoped) for his marathon journey, mornings and afternoons, was that he might have liked the ride back with his companions, or at least part of it. But it now sounded as though he hated it as much as we hated the thought of the waste of so much time.

This was only the beginning. A couple of days later he set off, perfectly fit again, to go back to school. He emerged from the bus in the afternoon, messy, groggy and very sorry for himself after a ghastly return journey. He had been sick three times, to the alarm of the mongol children and the elderly supervisor. This lady looked rather sternly at Pat—as if to imply we should never have got him into this jam.

It was difficult to know what to do. The educational psychologist at H told us that the headmaster at T had declared himself very pleased with the progress John had made; so much so, that he was himself considering which nearby school would be best to transfer him to; John needed to be stretched further, while he obviously still needed individual attention. Meanwhile, of course, we had been told by J. that the purpose of the unit at T was being changed. But we like to think that the headmaster's view that John should be transferred was taken in his best interests.

We ourselves were now desperately anxious for John to change school. But where?

Pat was in touch with the H educational psychologist every week. Each time she spoke to this lady she was aware of a genuine concern, at the other end of the line, to do something for John. Putting the receiver down, it was impossible not to believe that now, at last, the corner was about to be turned. The social worker was going to talk to the headmaster, and they would make a decision. A week later she would report that the headmaster was still thinking things over carefully, and that he wanted a discussion with us. Had we heard from him yet? No? Well, it wouldn't be long. . . . A week later, 'Heavens, this is dragging along, I agree. Well, I'll be that way tomorrow, and I'll make a point of seeing him. . . .'

By then, however, John had expressed his dislike of being treated like a long-distance parcel by being sick. Pat kept him home, took him to the doctor and talked over the problem with him.

Our doctor did not take long to make up his mind. He wrote a letter immediately to the authorities at H. He said that the school journey was having a bad effect on John's health; that it was a matter of importance that other arrangements should be made, either for his travel or for his schooling.

This had the effect of the educational psychologist at H ringing us. What a great shame, she declared, that everything took so long to fix. Had the headmaster at T been through to us yet, to make a definite suggestion? No? Well, she would certainly call on him in two days' time. . . .

'John mustn't do that journey any more,' Pat said to me after a day of no further news.

'If we keep him away from school,' I said, 'they can let him slip quietly out of their responsibility. Perhaps that's what they want.'

'I see that. But the doctor was *right*—he didn't say that just to please us. J. is picking him up herself from the centre, when she can—but it's costing her a lot in petrol, and she just can't go on like that.'

'What about the headmaster? Haven't you rung him?'

Pat glared at me. This was a sore point. Each time she tried to ring him she was unable to get past his secretary. 'And if you think I've got the time to sit around at the telephone all morning. . . .'

This was unanswerable: she hadn't. Simon was six months old, mercifully quiet at night, but inclined to scream the house down every second day. Louise spent three mornings a week at a kindergarten, but she still had to be taken there and collected. Pat was very tired, and the edginess that got into both our voices reminded me of the all-time low in the month before John's diagnosis.

'I'll tell you what,' I suddenly said. 'We'll step up the pressure.'

'How?' Pat demanded disbelievingly. Left to herself she would have tried each of the local newspapers, then the 'crusading' national dailies in turn. Soon afterwards a demonstration at the Houses of Parliament (camera teams from both BBC and ITV would have been specially invited). Though the temptation has been great, I've always felt this kind of thing would be more likely to spoil things for John at his *next* school, whatever he gained in the short term. Teachers, schools, local authorities—all tend to stick together against pressure on one of them from outside.

'For a start,' I declared, without further thought, 'I'll ring up Miss —— now.' (Because she sometimes worked at home, we had been given her home number by the H office.)

'But it's half past seven.'

'So it's half past seven! I'll ask if she's had supper.'

On the phone she discussed the possibility of getting someone to visit John as a home tutor. This did not appeal: if a child is autistic, we argued, he surely needs more experience of other children, in classrooms and playgrounds, not less. But if this were supplemented by visits to a primary school for part of the week we agreed it might do as a second best.

'What will you do then?' I asked the educational psychologist.

'There's one school—an ESN school—that might take him part time. Or there's the primary you mentioned at C. I'll have another talk with the headmaster at T and then get in touch with them.'

She was a bit surprised when I rang again the following evening. It was half past seven again, and I asked her what progress she had made. The third evening, she was half expecting my call.

'Could you please ring the headmaster at S?' she asked me. 'He now knows a bit about John, and he's expecting you to make an appointment to see him. He has a unit for young disturbed children at his school (which is ESN), and there's a boy there now who was thought to be autistic some time ago. The head's absolutely marvellous with children. There've been some astonishing cases of improvement there. And the main thing is, all his children seem to be very busy and happy.'

'It sounds fine,' I said, hardly believing my ears.

'Just one thing,' she added. 'He's very busy, and he sometimes seems a bit short on the telephone. . . .'

I hadn't made this part of the message entirely clear to Pat. When I came home the following evening she looked very dubiously at me.

It was the fourth evening that I was ringing the psychologist. We got along rather well now. 'Oh yes,' she said brightly. 'Well, I told you! You see he prefers children, I think. Anyway, he's perhaps the best headmaster I know, but he *can* seem a bit short sometimes. Do go ahead and see him.'

We visited him together. He was a bit doubtful about John going there so young. At just six years old, he would be the youngest in the 'unit' class. But he admitted John compared well with many of the others in size. Then he demanded to know what we were expecting that he would learn at S. What kind of result, exactly, were we looking forward to?

It's not an easy question at the best of times. It's much easier to talk of specifics: to say we want him to understand that roads, bridges and cliffs are dangerous; that some people will be friendly, while others won't; that certain kinds of games, certain kinds of hobbies, certain kinds of study and conversation can be fun. We could also say, truthfully, that we wanted him to be able to read and write, to enjoy both, and to understand what he was doing. And if he should catch up with other boys, we would like him to find out which sort of learning or skill he had the best aptitude for—maths, or music, or chemistry, or making model aeroplanes—and then do his best in them, taking examinations if it seemed reasonable. The question is difficult to answer because, in the end, we want to give him the moon. The best doesn't seem good enough.

I can't remember what our joint answer was. It was most likely an incoherent mixture of all the above paragraph.

The headmaster made no comment. Then he said he had not received any details about John from his counterpart at T. We filled in as best we could whatever the psychologist had not had time to tell him.

We were shown the unit classroom and were introduced to the teacher. Both seemed splendid.

All the more distressing then, when I rang the headmaster the next day, to be told by him, bluntly, that he would not take John. I asked him if he knew any other schools that might be right. He said no.

I took Pat out to dinner that evening, to compensate a little. It was a psychological mistake, actually, as it only served to focus our whole attention on the emptiness that should have been John's education.

'Let's ring up the secretary of the National Society,' Pat said after a long silence, 'and find out whether there are any cities in the British Isles where John would be better off.'

'There aren't any as far as I can see,' I murmured into my coffee. 'I might be able to get a job in New York, or Los Angeles. . . .'

Pat's imitation of an enthusiastic look made me drop this line entirely. (I could see her automatically thinking of riots, hoodlums, endless concrete, enormous medical and dental bills, alcoholics and tasteless food.)

I was soon on to the educational psychologist again. While agreeing that we should be trying other schools, she applied for another appointment at S and got one. 'This time,' she advised us, 'do try to look less academic. Don't say *anything* about examinations. And forget about psychology.'

Thus armed, we entered the head's study again. It was a very difficult decision, he told us. Our son was not quite this, not quite that. People had been telling him that finding the right school was very difficult; that even if we moved house, there was no guarantee of getting him into anywhere suitable. This was why we were having a second meeting.

'You haven't seen many of the children here, have you, Mr Rowlands?' he went on. 'There's quite a mixture, you know. Of course all kids are a mixture, but it might not be quite what you're expecting. . . .' He strode outside and asked for two boys to be sent in from the unit class. They came in separately, for a few minutes each. The first boy was smiling, and obviously aware that he was doing something a bit out of the ordinary. He was very eager to please—but his answers to some very simple questions suggested that he did not know how. The second boy was shy, and unwilling to look into anybody's eyes. I thought of John. But this boy's answers, although they were in whispers, showed that he knew a great deal about what was going on. We wondered what sort of emotions were getting in his way. When both boys had gone, the headmaster carefully scanned our faces for evidence of distaste, depression or disappointment with his school. Simultaneously he asked—what did we expect John to derive out of S school.

The interviews with the boys had shown us that whatever their problems were they had a strong combination of liking and regard for the headmaster—not awe, but the kind of eagerness to try to do what they felt he wanted from them. This was more impressive than their obvious disabilities.

I answered that whatever he felt was the best way of teaching these children was good enough for us.

'He's not going to be doing any reading or writing, you realize,' he said with his head inclined doubtfully on one side.

'If he's learning to get on with others, and take an interest in doing things for himself, that's all right by us,' I said firmly.

At this point he decided he might be indulgent. 'After a while (and it's got to be a good long while, mind you), we'll have another talk about John and see how we might co-operate in doing things for him. But first we need to find out what he's like for *ourselves*.'

Pat asked, hesitantly, 'Do you—are you taking him then?'

He spread his hands out, and told us that whatever we might suspect about pressure from local authorities he had had every intention from the outset of accepting John. He —and we—had needed time, however.

He came perilously close to being seized behind his desk at that moment, and being hugged. As it was, Pat restricted herself to bursting into tears.

To bridge the rather difficult gap of silence after this the headmaster informed us that he did not like psychiatrists coming round every ten minutes and checking on progress. We nodded vigorously.

Term was practically over, and we now had an impatient wait for the summer term. During the Easter holidays John made little headway with talking, but he did a lot of singing. The music therapist told us that we'd been rather absurd giving him French songs, or the more difficult or meaningless English songs. We would have done better to keep with 'Here we go round the mulberry bush', with its verses about 'This is the way we wash our hands', etc., accompanied by the right actions. This would have kept him closer to common words, to things that he actually did. There weren't many such songs, we objected. But she rounded on us, 'You're intelligent people—make some up!' Accordingly, we had invented for 'Row, row, row the boat' (which meant nothing to John):

Drive, drive, drive the car
Quickly through the rain.
Stop it a minute
And let me get in it,
And drive it off again.

Similarly for 'Kookaburra sits in the old gum-tree':

The black cat sits in the apple tree
Watching the birds very wickedly
Run—down the garden
Run—down the garden
Job is after me.

By choosing appropriate moments to sing these songs with John, Pat got him to understand their point. There was a limit, however, to the number of times I could stand listening to 'Drive, drive, drive the car' during the Easter holiday. 'Oh, John!' I said, exasperated, and for no logical reason, 'go and play it on the piano.' Solemnly he went to the piano and raised the lid. It took him about five goes to pick out the tune with his finger. He used only white notes, and took liberties with the time—but he kept the rhythm very well.

It was tempting to think that we could have built on this—eventually getting him to learn the piano by ear. But we knew from the therapist that the piano is a difficult instrument for *most* children. Also, we thought we should play according to the new headmaster's rules, and leave teaching to the school for a while.

He went off the piano after a few weeks. Maybe it's a missed opportunity, but we haven't tried to coax him back. He will probably come back in his own good time.

He also discovered he could whistle. This annoyed Louise, who found she could make whistling sounds but could not spin out a whole tune. It also annoyed me, because John started to search me out for joint whistling sessions. He would whistle the first bars of a tune, several times over, and come up close to me. Watching my mouth fixedly, he continued whistling the first part until I consented to join him in going through the whole piece. It was nice the first few times—infuriating the fifty-first time.

When he was told he was going to school again, at the beginning of the summer term, he said, 'No school! Bye-bye, school!' He was very distrustful of the plain green blazer we had bought him. When the bus appeared he had almost to be carried on board. Pat went with him to make sure the first day wouldn't be an utter disaster. In fact she needn't have bothered. Once he was actually there he was soon caught up in the stream of what was going on.

Two big changes happened very quickly. He was no longer alarmed by the bus coming in the morning. A bit resentful perhaps, but not alarmed. And in the afternoon, getting off the bus, he was as often as not cheerful, glad to be back but pleased (so it seemed) at having had a good day. What a difference from his pale shuffle off the step of the coach from the training centre!

The other boys in his new bus seemed to take to him. Cries of 'Hallo, Johnnie!' and 'Come and sit here!' came down the gangway when the door was opened for him.

Sometimes I pass the training centre coach when I go to the station on foot in the morning. Although it no longer stopped for John I used to go on waving to the old lady who sat in front, and the large, cheery mongol boys in the back. But I ceased meaning anything to the boys as soon as I was no longer someone who put a companion onto their coach. They look vacantly past me now as their world passes me by.

How splendid it would be to say, now that he's at the right school, the mists are clearing, and he's going to live happily ever after. Obviously this would be too much to hope for, even with a completely normal boy. There are so many different things involved. But we certainly believe that this step has at least given him a better chance of getting on even terms with life.

We have avoided pestering the people at S school with questions about what they are doing with John, and so on. This was part of our undertaking to the headmaster. In due course he kept his side of the bargain by volunteering information, when he felt that he and John's teacher had had enough experience of him to start forming opinions. Before the end of the first term we were invited over to have a thorough discussion about him—what he was good at, where his problems lay and how we might help him at home.

Meanwhile we had stopped any kind of teaching at home, except for two things, which certainly can't be called formal instruction. We did encourage John to say sentences instead of simply nouns. He has always to repeat what you say to him—either as an answer or instead of answering at all. An early type of conversation with him was like this:

'Do you want this, John?'

'This, John.'

'Do you want this chocolate?'

'Chocolate.'

(He might, by this time, be using his hands to get it.) Later on, the conversation became:

'Do you want this, John?'

'Do you want this, John?'

—and you got back exactly what you gave.

What we now found we could do, by trial and error, was to help him get further than this by saying *both* our part of the conversation and his. Soon, in simple situations, he no longer needed us to suggest his answer first. Moreover, and this was a real thrill when we first realized it, he learned to *vary* his answers, according to what he wanted. The conversation could now go:

'Do you want something, John?'

—followed by *either*

'I want an apple, please.'

or 'I want some chocolate, please.'

We got into the habit of saying to him, when we got into the car together, 'Where are we going, John? We're going to the shops!' Then we would repeat, 'Where are we going, John?' And he could tell us. Soon we could ask, 'Where are we going?' This seemed to make him consider what he was doing, rather than being simply a tourist. 'We're going to the—' (pause) '—back home!' Gradually he began to get it right too.

We've got no illusions that it's all our work. His improvement in using language is very much a matter of going to school, where he gets a lot of careful interest and skilled attention, and where there are lots of other children making conversational demands on him.

The other thing we've done is to read books or magazines with him—if he asks. He often doesn't want to for some time. Then he may get reminded about reading by seeing Louise concentrating hard on Orlando or Paddington Bear. At this he will seize something—usually a book he already knows and likes well—and cry, 'I want to read it, please! Read it please!'

Sometimes he seems to want us to do the reading, sometimes to work at it himself. We follow his wishes entirely. He particularly likes pointing at the picture side of the page, and saying what he knows is right for that part of the story. This is almost always a phrase that appeals to him, and that he likes repeating out of the context of the book. 'Poor Babar! He's crying!' is practically inevitable, whenever we come to the bit where the baby elephant becomes an orphan. John knows what crying means, and he likes to remind us that he does. He imitates crying sometimes—although he is grinning from ear to ear.

In the past year John has shown a definite preference for those books in the nursery that he can understand better, and which enable him to make more of these 'running commentary' observations. This is quite different from before, when he was indiscriminate.

A favourite with him has been Miss Moppet—below his age in interest, but above in reading standard. For a whole month he insisted on reading to us every day. We have tried to examine what makes a successful book in his eyes.

These, I think, are the main ingredients that help Miss Moppet hit the top of the charts: first, there are only two characters (Miss Moppet and the Mouse), who are *easy to identify*; second, there is a *simple plot* that develops *in small stages*, page by page; third, the plot is wholly a matter of actions, and doesn't for a moment depend on spoken words or thoughts; fourth, all the actions can easily be imitated, or demonstrated, to make the story clearer; and, finally, it is *short*, so that John's momentum is continued right the way through to the end.

I very much liked slipping into his room, on summer evenings, to see him looking through Miss Moppet again, after reading it to me earlier. He went back to the book for the personal pleasure it gave him. Again—few children *don't* do this sometimes. But our standard of comparison is the time when he would rub a friction toy up and down, up and down on the floor.

For every book like Miss Moppet, there are at least five which don't work. There doesn't seem to have been any great improvement in reading matter for children like John since Beatrix Potter wrote over fifty years ago.

Waiting for news about John's progress at school meant a lot of speculation on our part about what was going on there—whether he was making friends, what things he was enjoying, and so on. Once at the office, when I stopped and wondered what he was doing, I thought how nice it would be to hire a helicopter, to hover over the playground at break, to see the children come out, chat, form groups, play games. It might not reveal much, but it would show how John fitted in. Asking John a direct question got us no answer. We would just get the same words played back—because this was conversation that we could not help him develop.

'What were you doing at school, John?'

'What were you doing at school, John?'

It was good that he was smiling, though, at the words about school.

The next term Louise began school herself. When she came back in the afternoons she told Pat *everything*: about the girls who made too much noise; the hamster who got out of his cage; the dolls' tea-party in the Wendy-house. There was always something that had intrigued or delighted her.

John listened in to her eager reports. To help him feel one of the party Pat would break through Louise's patter, at least once, to ask, 'And did *you* have a good time at school today, John?'

No answers—until, one afternoon, John replied, 'Did you fall over in the playground?'

Pat quickly thought back to what Louise had been saying.

She was pretty sure that neither 'falling over' nor 'playground' had been mentioned. He was not just repeating something, he was contributing. When I came home from work it was the first thing I was told about. Had he won a scholarship I couldn't have been more pleased.

In a sense, it didn't matter two hoots whether or not he actually *had* fallen over in the playground—he had worked out a perfectly reasonable answer for us. But we were curious about how much was reality and how much was imagination. Pat had a good look at his knees when he got into the bath to see if there were any tell-tale bruises. There was a small bruise, in fact, but it didn't prove anything. How could we expect anyone at his school to have the slightest recollection of it?

Pat didn't receive much more information for a while, but one day:

'David bit me. Naughty David.'

When she took John up to the bus door next morning Pat simply had to ask the others, 'Does anybody know if a boy called David gave John a bite yesterday?'

Blank, amazed stares.

'I mean—it's not that we mind,' Pat explained to the bus, 'but we just want to know.'

One boy helped her out. 'David is John's friend,' he announced.

'He is? Oh—good!'

She gave the bus door a slam, realizing that the driver at least must think by now that she was completely out of her mind.

'There is a David,' she told me excitedly that evening. 'He's John's friend.'

'Is he really? Super!' I wanted to tell the story to everyone at work. But it takes at least five minutes, if you have to explain everything first.

Not long afterwards Pat had a chance to talk to John's teacher, when she went to the school to attend his medical exam. The teacher smiled at the story and saw the point of it at once. 'Actually,' she commented, 'you should have seen David. We had to rescue him from John.'

Chapter Eleven

John now, at seven, wants to tell us about a lot of things. But he's not sure about two points. What exactly *should* he say to us? And—what words should he use?

He hovers when Louise is saying things and getting replies. It's obviously a good thing to do. He'd like some of that, he feels. Sometimes he can cut in by repeating something we say that he recognizes, perhaps by elaborating it. If Louise talks about the swimming-pool at her school, he picks up a key word. 'Splash!' he shouts with a grin, waving his arms. '*Down* in the water. Splash!'

I turn to him and smile back. 'You like the swimming-pool, John? You like going splash in the water?'

He repeats his words again.

I go back to Louise, who has started talking about something else.

Suddenly John will try again, with 'Splash! All wet. Give me a towel, please!' And when he sees me looking at him he pretends to be lifting a towel from a rack.

It makes me remember how we had almost despaired of his ever being able to say anything that made sense. If there is one thing for which we feel particularly thankful towards his present school, it is that they have helped John to enjoy conversation. We are very anxious not to let him get discouraged in this. But the strain of following him down a single track, splashing on in swimming-pools when Louise has charged ahead, sometimes defeats our patience.

If he goes on wanting to join in what we're doing it seems to us that there must be so much more that he can achieve, given time. Wanting to talk with people is like a cornerstone to everything else. So we say to him, when we go to the shops, 'Can you see the toyshop, John?' As we're right next to it, he can't go wrong by pointing and replying, 'There's the toyshop.' If we stop, he might add, 'There's the toys.' Sometimes he reverts to an earlier stage of talking by repeating our words himself: 'See the toyshop, John.' We never suggest that he's wrong; after all, anybody can get distracted. We go on to point out different toys to each other in the window. He gets the words right for most of them now. He shows more interest in some than in others, which suggests choice.

One important discovery made it much easier for us to enjoy this kind of conversation. It is simply that passers-by, except perhaps for a very few, take absolutely no notice of it. Three years ago, when getting him to leave the swing doors of Boots' required brute force, I was convinced that everyone, but everyone, had stopped what they were doing, turned and were staring at us in amazement. It takes time to realize that people are not like that. Even if they do notice, they don't give a damn.

Two things about our toyshop conversations might surprise people—if they bothered to let themselves be surprised. I can't ask John, 'Which do you like best?' Similarly, I can't ask, 'What would you like to buy?' Choices are still very difficult for him, even when it's a matter of taking either of two fruit from a bowl. Verbal choices are even more difficult. He's very unsure about general words, like 'best', that you can't put a shape or a colour to. 'Buying' is a concept we haven't bothered to try to explain. He has a practical idea of what has to happen in a shop, but not much more. When the bread shop is quiet, we ask him to say to the assistant, 'One large white loaf, please,' or whatever. He has the money put into his hand. He passes the coins across, and accepts the change he is given. It's a pattern he enjoys, but the thought of saving or counting money, or calculating costs, is far away still.

Why he doesn't demand toys from the toyshop is an interesting question. I think it's because he has latched on to two important influences and watches them very closely. These help him to make some sense of the world, but restrict his view of what he could aim at. It's a bit like a sailor recognizing only two constellations in the sky—the Great Bear and the Little Bear. Anxious not to miss them, he doesn't let them out of his sight, changing his course according to them alone. So doing, he misses the richness that the rest of the sky has to offer. The rest, to him, is simply night. In John's case, the Great Bear is the children at school, and the Little Bear, with the Pole Star, is Louise. Whatever they are doing, provided it's not too difficult or alarming, is right. If he can watch them asking for things in shops long enough and consistently enough he will copy them, then understand what they are doing.

Louise decides to play at houses. Fine. This is what you do, then, at this time of day. She wants to spread this old sheet over the back of the bench in the garden. You take the end, then, and help her. Now she's taking her teddy-bear outside, to park him in her new house. You get yours, then, too. And so it goes on.

This way, he has learnt, he doesn't get left behind and he doesn't get bored. Out of the corner of his eye he may well notice that his parents like seeing him playing with Louise. He doesn't want to beat her, or to do anything better than she does—he just wants to join in.

I haven't seen him at school myself. But Pat, who went to the school Christmas party, says it's much the same. John hadn't experienced a school party before, but he knew how to mix in with the others, how to take their lead, how to enjoy himself. And—all credit to his teacher and to the headmaster—he seems to have learnt to take cues from teachers, much as the other children do.

This is partly, I feel, why he doesn't ask for ice-cream if we're passing the ice-cream shop. If he sees other children getting them though (and in particular, Louise), he tells us he wants one too.

Pat and I were always wary of his birthday parties. Usually Pat asked just a few children over that he knows reasonably well, given that he didn't like noisy, complicated crowds. Even so, at these parties, no one would have described him as particularly welcoming. Presents were put into his hands, and he watched them being unwrapped with complete indifference. The other children could play with them if they wanted. He tolerated games—but was relieved when it was tea time, or if we turned the party into a sing-song, or a percussion band session.

For his seventh birthday Pat asked the headmaster at S for the names and addresses of some of his friends at school, so that they could be invited along. There was also a nucleus of children he'd known for some time.

Three schoolmates turned up, together with Victoria, Alexander her brother and Alastair and Fiona from up the road. Louise, of course, was on the programme committee.

For the first time John seemed to be looking forward to the event. 'It's your birthday, soon', we told him; 'you're going to have a party. Happy birthday, John!' His smile got bigger each time. The words actually meant something without knowing exactly what (he suspected it was something good, that other children enjoyed). He was excited by the time the doorbell rang, and Victoria grinned at him on the doorstep.

Years ago he had utterly ignored what she had to offer. Now he was taking his present from her, saying, 'That's a present. Present for John.' He was looking forward to seeing what was inside.

'What do you say, John?' Pat murmured.

'Thank you—Victoria,' he declared. His hands were plucking with more eagerness than method at the string and the Sellotape. At last the wrapping yielded to him.

'What is it?' Alexander wanted to know. (He had forgotten.)

'That's a tractor,' John told him before anyone else.

Victoria looked pleased.

His school friends were all rather older than he was, but they seemed to enjoy the simple games we arranged as much as anybody. Each made a point of coming over to John every now and then, talking to him or helping him back into a game he'd lost track of. They took it in turns to be John's helper. (In 'Grandmother's Footsteps', for example, he needed a special signal to stop moving forward when the 'target' turned his head.) At first I thought they were just being on their best behaviour towards John, but their friendliness didn't stop when we left the room.

John was an active member of the whole party this time. He didn't win any prizes—because he didn't try to. But he found his share of the sweets hidden in the garden during the treasure hunt; he took his turn at throwing a football at the others' legs when they stood in a ring; he ran the gauntlet of 'British Bulldogs', and caught one or two when he himself was a 'Bulldog'. 'Passing-the-parcel' amused him: while most children have a compulsion to cheat at this game, he obeyed all instructions without showing the slightest desire to hold on to the parcel for longer than allowed. 'Musical Bumps' delighted him. He may well never win at this, because he takes his cue to 'bump' from the other children, not from the music. But he came a good third.

In short, he had a whale of a time.

He gets some invitations to other parties now too, not nearly as many as Louise, whose social life seems endless, but enough to make us feel that other parents are less embarrassed by him, and that other children are asking for him too.

When I went to collect him from Trevor's party one Saturday afternoon he was watching a film show with the others. Donald Duck was making him laugh, not so quickly or so often as the other children, but with the same pleasure.

What delighted me was Trevor leaving the room as soon as he saw me in the doorway. He was excited. 'I was talking to John,' he said, 'and he *talked back* to me!'

Not long ago it was difficult to imagine children outside the family taking the slightest trouble to make any contact with him.

If we go to an hotel now, or to a teashop at the week-end, we worry more about Simon than about John. If Simon is in a good mood—which is by no means predictable, because he is only one—we settle back and glance round continually. The other people will probably be looking at Simon, who is blond, blue-eyed and like a Mabel Lucie Attwell child. They may look at John, but they don't stop and scrutinize him. Nor do they look away from him hurriedly. This is what we really enjoy—their simply accepting him as one of the children in our party.

Some things, however, still mark him out as different. If someone asks him a direct question, using words in an order he doesn't recognize, he will just be silent. 'Perhaps he's shy,' is still the most obvious thing for them to say to themselves.

In case of emergency we had a St Christopher medal made

for him, which fits on a chain round his neck. Only a small stretch of chain is visible, so it doesn't make him obviously 'tagged'. One side of the medal has his name, address and telephone number on it. But we also taught him a little catechism—for use in case of need:

'What's your name?'

'John Rowlands.'

'Where do you live?'

'53 Top Meadow, Highmansbury.'

'What's your telephone number?'

'852417.'

In a crisis he should be able to reproduce enough of this conversation for people to help him. We only hope the system never needs to be tested.

Sometimes he makes engine noises, or whistles, at times when no one expects it. Many engine noises give him pleasure, and it makes me wonder if he reacts to them in the same way he does to music—because he likes the repetitive 'melody', or the constant rhythm.

People are more taken aback by the way he gets alarmed by little things that would mean nothing to most children. If our kettle is allowed to whistle for more than a moment he may scream. Cars with squeaky brakes are very unpleasant for him; against this, there is very little we can do. Birds don't worry him as they used to. Simon's crying can make him whimper—but this is a more complicated problem than dislike of a nasty noise. John likes Simon very much indeed, and seems as much distressed by the fact of his crying as by the sound of it. 'Pick him up, please!' John tells us when Simon starts off in earnest. When nothing seems to work, and Simon needs to be taken upstairs to his cot, John says, 'I want to turn the Simon off, please!' We have a lot of sympathy for him. 'So do we, John.'

More extreme is his fear of certain animals. Cats he loves—for which Bristol and Job must take much credit. He picks Job up gently, strokes him, puts him in his basket, feeds him. But if a dog approaches us when we are out walking on the common he gets very worried. He whimpers, goes pale and repeats softly what we have told him before—'Nice dog. He's all right. He won't hurt you'—as if these were magic phrases for spiriting dogs away. We need an aerosol spray to discourage dogs when we're on a walk.

One obvious answer is that we should keep a dog ourselves. Maybe we will, despite the cost in terms of nerves, and although Louise is the only one who wants one. (I can't think that Job really wants a dog, even for stalking practice.) It might get John used to dogs, at the very least. Possibly he will even realize that they can be treated as friends.

But at the moment we are concentrating on ponies. We can't afford to own one, but we can get him a riding lesson once a week. A surly, but pleasant-minded animal called Doyng submits to being ridden by John, who gets enormous pleasure out of it. When John sets off with a stable girl holding the leading rein I sometimes ask him, 'What are you doing, John?' He tells me, 'I'm riding on a horse!' and he puts on the largest grin he can muster. He's much more confident now, and he can keep the pony going when the leading rein is released. Cantering is some way off, but it will come.

Watching John playing with Simon gives us a lot of pleasure, as well as more hope for the future. John noticed me amusing Simon by bouncing his teddy-bear up and down on the cot edge, and suddenly letting it fall off, on top of him. Very soon John got the habit of slipping out of his bed and continuing the game. He woke him up for it if necessary. Fortunately Simon is tough—he could never have enough of it.

Now that Simon is on his feet the two of them join forces fairly often. Usually John smiles and gets interested in something Simon is doing, and follows his lead, repeating it. But John does some leading too. He knows what appeals to his brother, and he can choose something to distract him from what he is doing and make him return to John.

If anything new or daring is involved we usually trace it to Simon. Fortunately for himself and for us, since he has absolutely no conception of road danger, John has never had an urge to wander, and so we have been spared a lot of anxiety. Lately we have come across John and Simon together, outside the gate, once thirty yards down the opposite side of the road. John lifts the latch, but the demon who suggests the plot must be Simon.

Simon is late talking but he understands most of what we tell him. Somehow he is communicating with John, often making complicated arrangements with him. This is wonderful—but we must get better at anticipating their brand of mischief.

To say John has no concept of danger would be overstating the case. Once he touches the outside of an oven, for instance, he avoids it carefully. But anything he hasn't learnt direct from experience might just as well not exist for him.

We stop at the kerb with him, gesture towards the traffic and say, solemnly, 'Very, very dangerous.' Although this is the same phrase that Pat has used for ovens, the steam-iron and electric points, he doesn't take us at all seriously. He repeats it, with emphasis, 'Very, *very* dangerous,' and laughs. We take him through the 'kerb drill', with more hope than faith. We murmur to ourselves, please, please let him understand gradually about traffic, without anything terrible having to happen first.

However much we loved him before, protecting him

seems even more important now that he is growing up and taking his place in the world. Over this last year he has shown us what enormous potential he has as a friend, both at home and elsewhere; how much more anxious he is to share his experiences, even if he can't find the right words; how much more likely he is to become someone who is useful, liked and respected.

There's a long way still to go, and sometimes I become gloomy about it. When John is older, other children of his age may be that much more cruel. When he reaches puberty there may be sexual problems to deal with. I don't always think this way, but the thoughts recur. Pat is more confident. She concentrates on specific problems.

For instance, he is now too old to be taken into the women's changing-rooms at the swimming-pool, but he would be terribly confused if he went alone into the men's. The same applies to public lavatories: he could probably manage perfectly well by himself in the Gents, but the kinds of approach that might be made to him are horrifying. All this means planning journeys and trips rather carefully.

When he was diagnosed, I still think the acid test question was, 'Will he ever get married?'

The consultant's 'No, I don't think so,' was a harsh verdict. This exchange hinted at far more than was actually said. It suggested he would not be capable of the kind of relationship on which a successful marriage can be based; that he would not be able to support a household; that we had better think about how, and by whom, his affairs would be looked after when he grew up; that he might be sexually frustrated.

Perhaps the consultant would say the same today. But we have much more cause now to be confident about John's future—even if he does fall short of becoming a suitable marriage partner. There is so much more contact now between him and us, that the prospect of looking after him does not seem anything like the life sentence that sometimes seemed to have been read out to us.

He talks to other children a little. We know now that he *will* have companions, even if they won't be bosom friends as most people understand it. He will talk to them a lot.

The consultant had also said something about John 'looking as though he would work his way through'. It has been proved true. He still has less of the initiative, less of the drive we see in other children. But he is determined, in his way. He is working his way through, and he will reach us.

The day I started this chapter Louise demonstrated proudly how she could swing upside-down on a rope ladder, hanging by her knees. Three days later, despite many bruises—so many that I tried to put him off—John got there, and he swung. His grin of pride was bigger than Louise's had been, and (perhaps we're wrong) we praised him rather more than his sister. After all, he is *working* his way through.

If Pat and I died tomorrow—we have to think of this, sometimes—there is a contingency plan. My oldest school friend has agreed to be the children's guardian. He has watched John growing up and, although we don't discuss it, I know he is less alarmed now than he might have been about John's possible entry into his family. Having other children, of course, makes us more confident about future crises.

Simon, still under two, thinks John is a super brother to play with, and probably hasn't started to compare him with anyone else. Louise's views are difficult to fathom. She asks us very little about him. She certainly understands more than she lets on.

The other day it was Pat's turn to drive Louise and the rest of the 'school run' to school in the morning. The girls were saying to each other how nice it was not to have to endure the company of the 'yuks' that day—i.e. some boys who are usually in the school run but had a holiday.

'I don't want any yuks in the car!' cried Sally.

Everyone agreed.

'Is your brother a yuk?' Clare asked Sally.

'Oh yes! He's a *terrible* yuk! He shouts a lot, he breaks my toys, he pushes me over, and—and he plays football in the dining-room.' She turned to Louise. 'What about John?'

Louise shook her head. As she was stopped at a traffic light Pat was able to look at her face in the driving mirror. She saw a very serious, thoughtful expression.

'No. John's not a yuk,' Louise declared.

'Why?' Sally and Clare demanded.

'Well . . . he's not so good at talking,' Louise told them. 'He's a bit slower than other boys.'

At least she doesn't seem to *worry* about John. She gets jealous of Simon, sometimes, and muses, 'Wouldn't it be nice just to have John and me!' While she gets justifiably annoyed with him at times (especially when he loses the tops off her felt-tip pens, or tickles her when she's drawing), she rounds on anyone who tells John off too sharply in her presence. When this happens she literally quivers with rage.

Gradually she will realize how John is different. She doesn't know the word 'autism'. If and when she asks, we will try to give her an idea of what it means. But she seems far too young to have her mind burdened with clinical details. It is no bad thing for her to accept that some people have John's handicap, and that this can be overcome if they are helped. At least one potential helper is not going to recoil with horror at mental handicap. We have little patience with other parents who seem to want to protect their children from having any close contact with John.

'What did you do at school today, John?' I like to ask him, when I get home.

'Did you play on the climbing frame?' he answers.

'On the climbing frame? Did you?'

'Did you do climbing?'

'What else did you do, John?'

'Naughty boy!'—with a large grin—'Did you pull David's hair?'

I get the picture. Poor old David! We went round to the school yesterday to speak to John's teacher and the headmaster at S. His teacher told us that John and David were still good friends; still had tremendous fights. She reassured us that John was as good for David as David was for John.

The headmaster told us off for admitting that we were 'excited' about the progress that John had made. If you get excited at progress, he told us, you get depressed at no progress. Therefore, he concluded, avoid emotional extremes. He relented to the extent of allowing us to feel pleased. And, of course, we are enormously pleased.

'Well, we haven't done anything really,' the headmaster continued. 'We haven't had any psychiatrists looking in. I don't think we *want* any of them looking in, do you?' He cocked a wary eyebrow at me.

I shook my head. 'Why disturb a winning combination?'

It's not easy to be precise about how the 'combination' has worked. The main components are, I believe, giving him individual attention some of the time, and drawing him, patiently but persistently, into what the class is doing for the rest of the time. And they observe carefully how he reacts to stimulation of different kinds.

The headmaster looked at me very seriously. 'There might

be quite a lot of kiddies like him, you know, who don't fit in. They get told they're lazy at home, or a nuisance. They go straight into the local primary because nobody sees that there's anything really wrong. There they sit with forty others who've got more go about them, and understand better what's being told them. After a bit it's not surprising they just retire into themselves.'

He is right, there must be many fugitive minds—that shy away to varying degrees. They miss the world, and they miss identification..

'Well, we haven't done anything, really.' The headmaster repeated this as we went out. We know what he means—no fancy techniques, and expecting John to fit in with the rest of the class for things like assembly, dinners, going here, going there and running errands. But, in another sense, he's quite wrong. What he and John's teacher have done is to accept John as an important individual, and to give him their time and their energy.

It's worth an awful lot of effort to find a place like S; and in this country, still, an awful lot of effort is needed to find one.

There is no system that infallibly organizes, provides for or even wonders about children like John. You have to work.

Postscript

It is nearly two years since I wrote the last chapter. John has not stood still. He is bigger and stronger for one thing. He is also sunnier, naughtier, more determined in his efforts to let us know what he feels and altogether more individual as a character.

He is more nimble with his fingers than we would have given him credit for. He enjoys making cut-out models, and recently brought back from school a magnificent cardboard tiger, with finely crimped whiskers. There are all sorts of kitchen jobs which he has now mastered, and he takes a pride in his work in the garden, and in cleaning and polishing the car.

His teacher reports that he is beginning to take an interest in writing. This may be a long, slow haul, but it will come in the end. Meanwhile he does not do a great deal of reading, but what he reads seems to have more *point*.

One helpful tip on reading has inspired Louise to great activity. After lunch at week-ends, instead of an automatic sweet distribution, she takes it on herself to write messages for the whole family, e.g.—'John—your sweet is on the window-sill in the kitchen'. Reading then becomes a kind of treasure hunt. John got the idea very quickly, and keeps his messages for hours after he has acted on them.

His younger brothers, Simon and (now) Stephen, tend to view this message business as a nuisance, but they get special help from their sister.

His riding is the most exciting part of the week for him. By luck, we found an excellent teacher, who has got him rising to the trot, cantering, turning and stopping the pony far more capably than I had imagined possible.

There are still areas where we could be doing better for him. We've done nothing about his resistance to swimming. We haven't bought a dog that he could learn to like. We haven't taken as much interest in his collection of oddities—from snail-shells to rubber-bands—as perhaps we should be doing.

There are also plenty of problems still to be faced. S may not be the best school for him right up to sixteen. Puberty may be a distinctly difficult time. And there is always the fear that somebody, somewhere, will take advantage of him.

But both Pat and I are much more hopeful now than we ever were. We don't feel we are having to chase a fugitive mind all the time. We know that when he does flit away he comes back. This makes us very proud of him.

Appendix

(a) What is an autistic child?

This is very difficult to answer in a few words. A typical autistic child has no obvious brain damage, and his sight, hearing and other senses appear intact. But, probably because of a subtle defect in his brain, he cannot perceive things properly. He fails to categorize and understand what he sees and hears. This makes it difficult for him to learn to talk; to relate to other people; to understand what they are saying and expecting of him; to make sense of what is going on; to distinguish between what is incidental, what is helpful, and what is dangerous; to build on his experience. And yet he is often intelligent. Sometimes he is very intelligent. His mind has a real potential, but seems fugitive, distracted. Such a child can develop behaviour problems, particularly when those who do not realize what is wrong try to force him to behave and grow up normally.

This is a very simplified picture. For one thing, there is a wide range of degrees of severity: the most heavily handicapped children seem, at first, very different from those who are mildly affected. There are also strong differences between those who are 'hyperactive' with their autism and those who are 'passive'. Some autistic children go through a hyperactive phase, in which they are perpetually on the move, looking round restlessly, and making all sorts of repetitive movements with their hands. Further, there is demonstrably less 'autism' noticeable among those who have received suitable training than among those who have not.

(b) *How is autism defined?*

Early infantile autism is a late arrival in textbooks on mental handicaps. A psychiatrist called Kanner first proposed that 'autism' was something that could be identified separately from other mental handicap or illness. This has been known as 'Kanner's Syndrome'. A situation soon developed in which the label 'autistic' tended to be applied without much discrimination, in hospitals and universities. In the 1950s therefore a working party was set up to investigate the evidence for the syndrome and, if possible, to define it.

They emerged with the 'Nine Points', which they concluded should characterize cases that might be classified as 'early infantile autism'. This has remained the basis for definition. The Nine Points cover the following characteristics:

1. Autistic children take a long time to start talking—and sometimes never do.

2. When they do talk, there are particular oddities in their speech—e.g. they mix up personal pronouns, etc.

3. They withdraw from contact with others—especially in surroundings that are foreign to them.

4. They use their senses differently—e.g. using peripheral vision; smelling and tasting things in order to get to know them, etc.

5. They move oddly, sometimes delighting in twisting or flapping movements with their hands.

6. Their reactions to heat, cold and pain are often unusual.

7. They have unpredictable moods, and are sometimes given to violent tantrums for little apparent reason.

8. They use objects in peculiar ways—e.g. obsessively playing with small toys, making meaningless collections—sometimes even suggesting that objects are more important to them than people.

9. Change is often resisted, or disliked—change of routine, of colour scheme, etc.

Not all of these are going to be observed in the same child at the same time. Naturally, practitioners vary in their attitudes about which of the Points are more significant than others.

More recent work by Dr Bernard Rimland, in which a computer was used to analyse data about a large number of autistic children, suggests that there may be several separate forms of 'autism'—possibly seven—each with several sub-groups. These differ partly in the symptoms that the children display, partly in their circumstances—e.g. onset at birth, or later; the kind of training that seems helpful, etc.

(c) *How does autism happen?*

The disclaimer in the Introduction had better be repeated at this point. I have no medical background whatever. Apart from a degree course in psychology, and my experience as a parent, I have no particular right to attempt an analysis of this kind.

There are four broad categories of reasons why children may become autistic, that are logically possible. These have been called A, B, C and D in the diagram on page 140. They are not mutually exclusive, although some combinations of reasons are much less likely than others.

A *Hereditary*. There is no body of evidence pointing to autism running in families, but certain racial groups seem

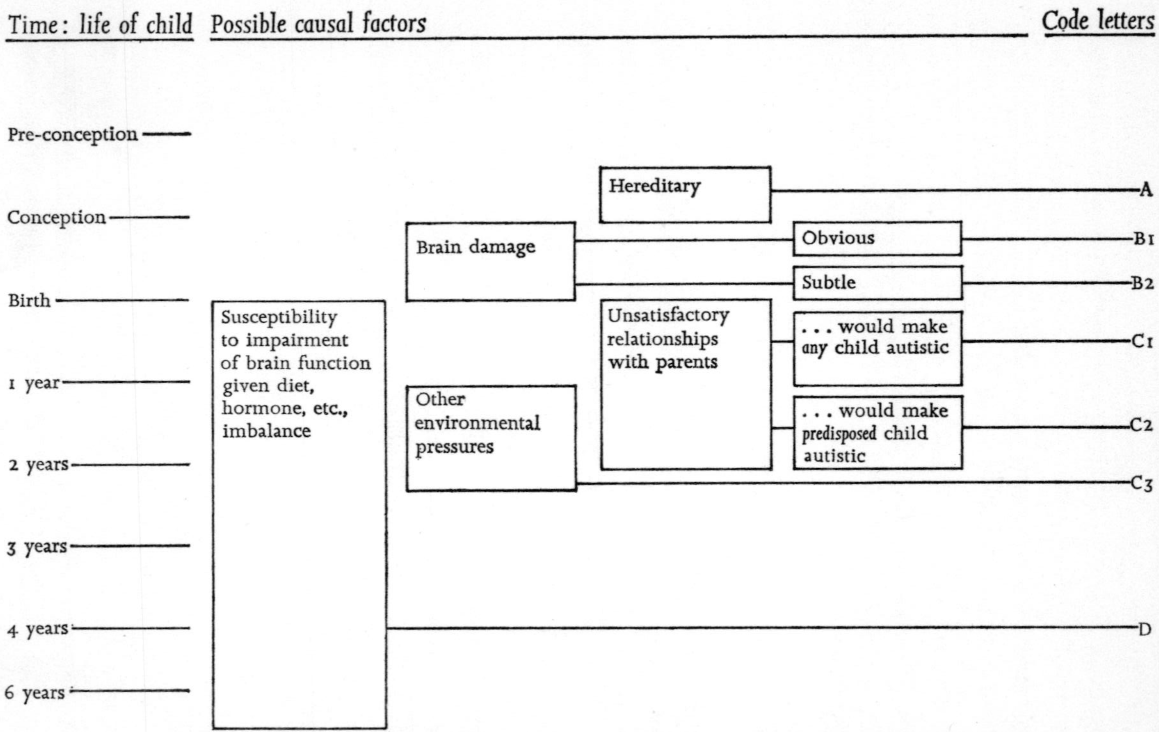

Factors that may cause, or contribute to, the onset of autism at different stages of development

more likely to have autistic children than others, e.g. there are more Anglo-Saxon and more Jewish autistic children than Latins or Slavs. Further, autistic children's parents tend to have had more education than the average population, or else to have specialist skills. Some researchers have noticed that these parents tend to be asthmatic. It is possible to inherit a predisposition, as opposed to autism itself.

B *Brain damage.* Many autistic children have no *obvious* brain damage, but the possibility of *subtle* brain damage is suggested by the characteristic oddities that autistic children show in their use of their senses. Nobody is sure what, exactly, this subtle damage could be, but the fact that autistic children tend to share physical characteristics could indicate that they share a brain imperfection as well (e.g. they are dark in complexion, and boys rather than girls, double-jointed, etc.).

C *Environment.* The first clinical observations made were taken as evidence of unsatisfactory relationships with parents. This stemmed partly from the fact that schizophrenia in children has often been imputed to this, and those who were now called autistic had sometimes been assumed to be schizophrenic. This theory is partly based on a feeling that the children are making a kind of choice, as if they were fleeing from overbearing parents, out of reality and into autism. It is hard to see how they could flee into some of the Nine Points, e.g. sense oddities, common speech peculiarities, etc., and harder still to see how they could choose to be boys, rather than girls, and to have symmetrical features.

A watered-down version of this theory makes parental or other environmental pressure a contributory, as opposed to a sole, cause.

D *Diet, hormone imbalance.* Any simple explanation of autism in terms of a metabolic problem, or a poison affecting the brain, seems most unlikely given that no such causal effect has yet been discovered. A more complex possibility is that some children have a predisposition towards autism which depends on some change in the chemistry of the brain for them to become autistic.

On the diagram, a time-scale shows roughly over what period a child may be susceptible to autism, if one of the causal factors applies. The fact that some children only seem to show autistic symptoms after several years' normal development seems to tell against C (or, at least, C1), and to suggest that D may be possible.

It should be repeated that certain combinations of causal factors are perfectly possible: e.g. A & B2 & D. This would make the time-scale a purely notional matter.

(d) *What can you do if you are told, or suspect, that your child is autistic?*

The first thing must be to get expert medical advice. Some doctors may never have come into contact with an autistic child at close quarters, but they can refer you to a specialist for a consultation, either privately, or under the National Health Service.

With very young children, a clear-cut diagnosis may not be possible immediately. But once it is agreed that your child is probably autistic, advice and information can be got from:

The Secretary
The National Society for Autistic Children
1a Golders Green Road
London NW11 8EA

This society is the only one, at present, to specialize in

promoting the interests of autistic children. But help and advice are also provided by the National Society for Mentally Handicapped Children, which has branches all over the country.

(e) *Are there any useful books to read?*

Here is a list of those books which I, as a parent, have found to be of practical value:

Autistic Children by Lorna Wing; National Association for Mental Health, 1964. Now superseded by her longer book, *Autistic Children—a Guide for Parents*; Constable & Co., 1971.

Infantile Autism by Bernard Rimland; New York, 1964, London, Methuen, 1965. (Obtainable from Medical Books (London) Ltd, 49 Newman St, London W1P 4BB)

Early Childhood Autism—Clinical, Educational, and Social Aspects, edited by J. K. Wing; Pergamon Press, 1966.

The Birth of Language—a Case History of a Non-verbal Child by Shulamit Kastein and Barbara Trace. Charles C. Thomas, Springfield, Illinois, 1966. (Obtainable from H. K. Lewis & Co., P.O. Box 66, 136 Gower Street, London WC1E 6BS)

Certain other books on the subject are worth recommending for their interest value:

The Wild Boy of Aveyron by Jean-Marc Gaspard Itard, trans. by George and Muriel Humphrey; New York, Appleton-Century-Croft, 1962.

The Siege by Clara Claiborne Park; New York, 1967, London, Colin Smythe, 1969.

The film based on *The Wild Boy of Aveyron*, *L'Enfant Sauvage* by François Truffaut, is a particularly sensitive and convincing account of the development of a very severely handicapped child. There are several useful documentary films that have been produced by television companies in the U.K. and abroad: the NSAC keeps a list of these, and can sometimes arrange for them to be borrowed and shown at private meetings.

Index